MEDITERRANEAN KETOGENIC DIET

REINVIGORATE YOUR BODY AND HAVE A HEALTHIER LIFESTYLE

MEDITERRANEAN KETO DIET FOR ALL FAMILY, LOSE WEIGHT AND IMPROVE YOUR MIND. COOKBOOK FOR BEGINNERS

Tilly Heather

Copyright © Tilly Heather

Editing by **Tilly Heather**

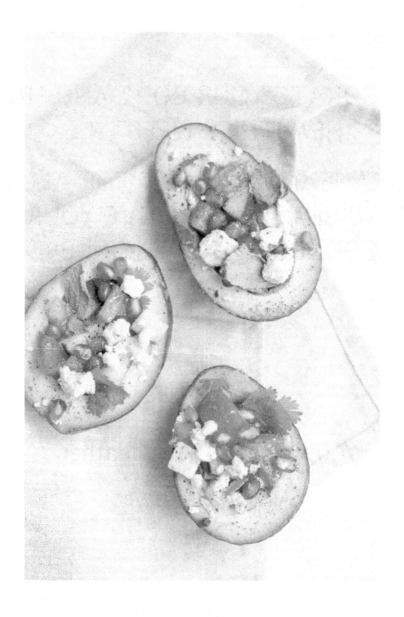

Table of Content

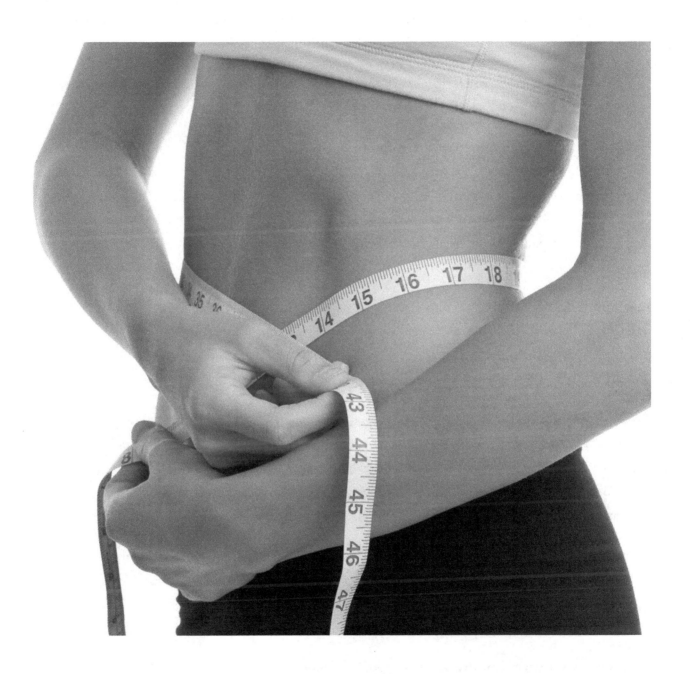

Chapter 1. Keto Cuisine

Keto nutritional strategy is to consume high fat, moderate amounts of protein, and minimal carbs. It will help your body enter into the ketosis state, thereby resulting in the ketone bodies' production. Your body will soon turn into a fat-burning machine, helping you achieve your goal weight.

Remember, fat is an essential macronutrient that plays a significant role in the ketogenic diet, and it is not the fact that it makes you fat!

Cut carbs. The first and most vital step to take towards the Keto diet is cutting out carbs. I know it may sound straightforward, even trivial, but it's as tougher as it seems for most of us. The majority of us may have bread, pasta, potatoes, rice, or something similar at least once a day, but in a Keto diet, that has to be avoided. As someone who loves pasta, this was incredibly hard for me, but I managed, which paid off. We need to stay below 50 grams of carbs per day, ideally, down to 20 grams per day.

Limit protein. Now that we've cut out carbs, we need to replace them with the fatty foods that will power us when we reach ketosis. Many people make the mistake of replacing their carbs with protein, which is an issue because excess protein can be converted into glucose. If we have extra protein in our diet, we may find it harder to reach ketosis.

Avoid sugar. This diet may be a high-fat diet, but it doesn't mean sugary foods are good for us. Glucose, fructose, and sucrose are all incredibly common in candy, soft drinks, and junk food that you come across. These sugars are the exact things that we are trying to remove by cutting our diet's carbs. Besides natural sugars, we should also avoid sweeteners like xylitol, maltitol, aspartame, and saccharin. These sweeteners have similar net carbs to table sugar and should be avoided all the same.

Keep your vegetables above ground! Vegetables are an essential part of Keto, but we need to include only above-ground vegetables. Root vegetables are high in starch and sugars, while the vast majority of green vegetables are light on carbs. Some of the best vegetables for Keto diet include lettuce, spinach, asparagus, avocado, cauliflower, cucumber, and tomato.

Be careful with what you drink. Many people overlook their drinks while making diet, but we won't make that same mistake. In Keto diet, the drinks you have during the day can make or break your path to ketosis. Luckily, we have plenty of healthy options when it comes to refreshments. We've all been taught since we were children that we should always drink plenty of water, and there isn't any reason for don't do that. Put slices of lemon or lime into your glass, and there you have a delicious drink with zero carbs. Tea and coffee are fantastic too, but avoid using any of the sugars or sweeteners mentioned above, and be careful using too much milk. Diet soft drinks can be fine as well, be careful to read the ingredients; many diet drinks may have sweeteners, which are still carb-heavy. Lastly, alcohol is very light on carbs; wine and pure spirits are all fine to drink in a Keto diet.

Increase healthy fats! As we've already read, the Keto diet is high-fat. As we've been taught to avoid fat for so many years, it is often hard to wrap our heads around needing more than 60% fat in our daily diet. Luckily, there are easy and healthy ways of increasing your fat intake. One tasty and easy to find a source of healthy fats is fish. Salmon, mackerel, herring, and sardines are great examples of fatty fish, all of which are easy to start and make for tasty meals. Another fantastic source of fats is oil. Coconut, avocado, and olive oil are healthy oil choices, which we can use for cooking meals and garnishing vegetables. Lastly, animal products are also a great way of filling out your healthy fats quota for the day. Eggs, cheese, butter, and cream can make perfect snacks throughout the day, especially when partnered with low carb nuts such as pecans, macadamias, and Brazil nuts.

Use a calorie counter. Even if you're following a detailed meal plan, keep a calorie counter with you. We must hold ourselves to the requirements of our Keto diet. Having an app or notepad that allows us to track our meals will help us learn more about our diet and reach our goals better.

New diets can be challenging initially, but the beauty about the Keto diet is that every change you need, makes it easily achievable. It's a series of small, manageable steps that lead to an incredible result. Take your time to work these changes into your daily life, and don't rush. Keto done at your own pace is the best kind of Keto.

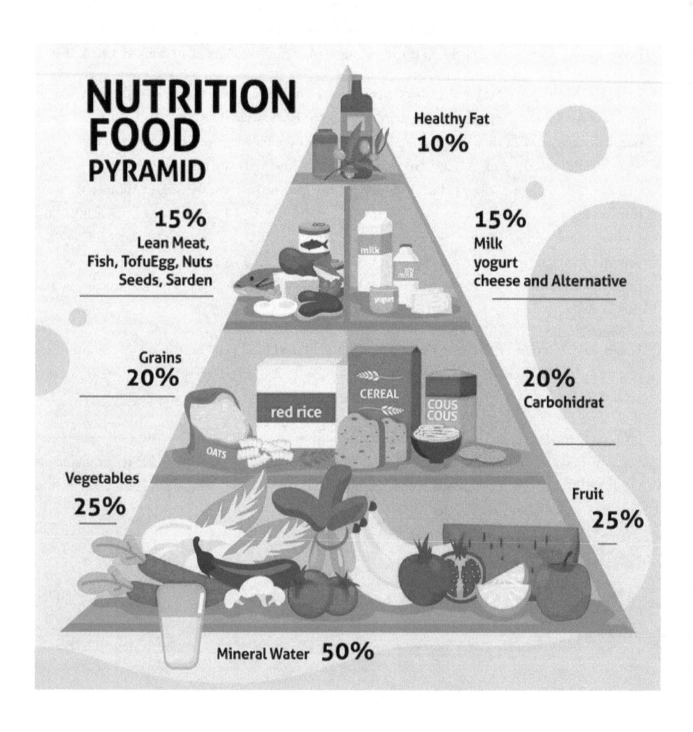

NUTRITION FOOD PYRAMID

Healthy Fat 10%

15% Lean Meat, Fish, TofuEgg, Nuts Seeds, Sarden

15% Milk yogurt cheese and Alternative

Grains 20%

20% Carbohidrat

Vegetables 25%

Fruit 25%

Mineral Water 50%

Best Foods to Fit into the Keto Diet for Older Adults

I will go over what food you should consider incorporating into your Keto diet. But the general guideline is that all foods that are nutritious and low in carbs are excellent options.

Seafood

Fishes and shellfishes are perfect for Keto diets. Many fishes are rich in B vitamins, potassium, as well as selenium. Salmon, sardines, mackerel, and other fatty fish also contain many omega-3 fats that help to regulate insulin levels. These are so low in carbs that it is negligible.

Shellfishes are a different story because some contain very few carbs, whereas others contain plenty. Shrimps and most crabs are good but beware of other types of shellfish.

Vegetables

Most vegetables contain a lot of nutrients that your body can greatly benefit from even though they are low in calories and carbs. Plus, some of them contain fiber, which helps with your bowel movement. Moreover, your body spends more energy breaking down and digesting food rich in fiber, so it helps with weight loss.

Cheese

Milk is not good, but you can get away with cheese, though. Cheese is delicious and nutritious. Thankfully, although hundreds of types of cheese are out there, all of them are low in carbs and full of fat. Eating cheese may even help your muscles and slow down aging.

Avocados

Avocados are so famous nowadays in the health community that people associate the word "health" to avocados. It is for an excellent reason because avocados are very healthy. They contain lots of vitamins and minerals, such as potassium. Moreover, avocados are shown to help the body go into ketosis faster.

Meat and Poultry

These two are the staple food in most Keto diets. Most of the Keto meals revolve around using these two ingredients. It is because they contain no carbs and contain plenty of vitamins and minerals. Moreover, they are a great source of protein.

Eggs

Eggs form the bulk of most food you will eat in a Keto diet because they are the most versatile food item. Even a large egg contains so little carbs but contains plenty of protein, making it a perfect Keto diet option.

Moreover, eggs are shown to have an appetite suppression effect, making you feel full for longer and regulating blood sugar levels. It leads to lower calorie intake for a day. Just make sure to eat the entire egg because the nutrients are in the yolk.

Coconut Oil

Coconut oil and other coconut-related products such as coconut milk and coconut powder are perfect for a Keto diet. Coconut oil, mainly, contains MCTs converted into ketones by the liver to be used as an immediate energy source.

Plain Greek Yogurt and Cottage Cheese

These two food items are rich in protein and a small number of carbs, small enough that you can safely include them into your Keto diet. They also help to suppress your appetite by making you feel full for longer. They can be eaten alone and are still delicious.

Olive Oil

Olive oil is very beneficial for your heart because it contains oleic acid that helps to decrease heart disease risk factors. Extra-virgin olive oil is also rich in antioxidants. The best thing is that olive oil can be used as a primary source of fat and has no carbs. The same goes for olive.

Nuts and Seeds

These are low in carbs but rich in fat. They are also healthy and have a lot of nutrients and fiber. They help to reduce heart disease, cancer, depression, and other risks of infections. The fiber in these also help to make you feel full for longer, so you would consume fewer calories, and your body would spend more calories digesting them.

Berries

Many fruits contain too many carbs that make them unsuitable in a Keto diet, but unlike berries, they are high in fiber and low in carbs. You may include the best berries in your diet, such as blackberries, blueberries, raspberries, and strawberries.

Butter and Cream

These two food items contain plenty of fat and a minimal amount of carbs, making them an excellent option to include in your Keto diet.

Shirataki Noodles

If you love noodles and pasta and don't want to give up on them, then shirataki noodles are the perfect alternative. They are rich in water content and contain a lot of fiber, which means low carbs and calories and hunger suppression.

Unsweetened Coffee and Tea

These two drinks are carb-free, so long as you don't add sugar, milk, or other sweeteners. Both contain caffeine that improves your metabolism and suppresses your appetite. A word of advice to those who love light coffee and tea lattes, though; they are made with non-fat milk and contain a lot of carbs.

Dark Chocolate and Cocoa Powder

These two food items are delicious and contain antioxidants. Dark chocolate is associated with the reduction of heart disease risk by lowering the blood pressure. Just make sure that you choose only dark chocolate with at least 70% cocoa solids.

Allowed Product List

If you've decided to go on the Keto diet after 50, be sure you won't regret your choice! So when you start something new, the first and the main thing you need to do is consult the Keto dietary features. Nevertheless, most importantly, you must look at the list of allowed products to remember this list and adhere strictly to it.

Don't worry! The low-carb eating plan isn't overly limited. Check out what products you can and must buy in the supermarket and start a new stage in your life.

Meat and Poultry

Chicken, beef, pork, lamb, turkey, veal includes no-carb, but high protein and fat intake. That is the primary reason why meat and poultry products are known as the staples for the Ketogenic diet. Besides this, bacon and organ meats are also allowed for consumption.

Seafood

When it comes to seafood, you also have an excellent list. You can buy and cook a lot of delicious dishes from:

Lobster, Shrimp, Octopus, Salmon, Tuna, Oysters, Mussels, Squid, and Scallops

The most useful Keto seafood is the crab and shrimp. They don't contain carbohydrates at all.

Vegetables

Only low-carb and non-starchy veggies can be eaten by people who go on the Keto diet. It means that you can add the following vegetables:

Avocados, Tomatoes, Cucumbers, Zucchini, Radishes, Mushrooms, Eggplant, Celery, Bell peppers, Herbs, Asparagus, Kohlrabi, Mustard, Spinach, Lettuce, Kale, and Brussels sprouts

Dairy Products

It would be best if you were careful with dairy. Not all dairy food can be useful for you if you want to stick to the Keto diet. Here are the products you can buy and cook:

Eggs, Butter and ghee, Heavy cream and whipping cream, Sour cream, Unflavored Greek yogurt, Cottage cheese, and Hard, semi-hard, soft, and cream cheeses

Berries

Unfortunately, most fruits have high levels of carbs and can't be included on the Keto diet. However, you can consume:

Blackberries, Raspberries, Strawberries, and Blueberries

Nuts and Seeds

A lot of experts recommend paying attention to nuts and seeds that are high-fat and low-carb. You can add such nuts and seeds to your dishes as:

Almond, Pecans, Walnuts, Hazelnuts, Brazil nuts, Pumpkin seeds, Sesame seeds, Chia seeds, and Flaxseed

Coconut and Olive Oils

To cook tasty fatty dishes, you need oil. Coconut and olive oils have unique properties that make them suitable for a Keto diet. These oils are rich in fat and boost ketone production. Moreover, they can be used for salad dressing and adding to cooked dishes.

Low-Carb Drinks

The Keto diet means that you should drink only unsweetened coffee and tea because they don't include carbs and fasten metabolism. Besides, you can drink dark chocolate and cocoa. Such drinks have low levels of carbohydrates, and that's why they're permitted.

Prohibited Product List

When it comes to food lists, you should avoid the low-carb, high-fat diet, be attentive, and check it carefully. Well, you can't eat:

- Grains (like oatmeal, pasta, bulgur, corn, wheat, buckwheat, rice, etc.)

- Low-fat dairy (fat-free yogurt, skim milk, skim Mozzarella, etc.)

- Most fruits (melon, watermelon, apples, peaches, bananas, grapes, oranges, plums, grapefruits, mangos, cherries, pineapples, pears, etc.)

- Starchy veggies (potatoes, beets, turnips, parsnips, etc.)

- Grain foods (pasta, popcorn, muesli, cereal, bagels, bread, etc.)

- Some oils (soya bean oil, grape seed oil, sunflower oil, peanut oil, canola oil)

- Typical snack foods (crackers, potato chips, etc.)

- Trans fats (margarine)

- Sweeteners and added sugars (corn syrup, cane sugar, honey, agave nectar, etc.)

- Sweetened drinks (sweetened coffee and tea, juice, soda, smoothies)

- Alcohol (sweet wines, cider, beer, etc.)

Chapter 3. Recipes from Italy

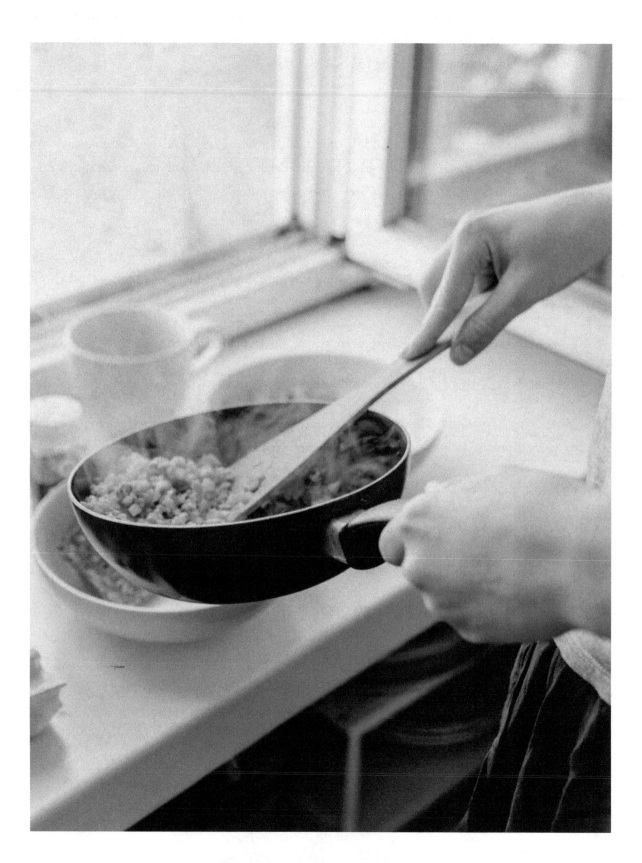

Spinach and Red Pepper Frittata

Preparation Time: 5 minutes

Cooking Time: 22 minutes

Servings: 8

Ingredients:

- 8 eggs
- 1/3 cup of heavy whipping cream
- ½ cup of shredded cheddar cheese
- ¼ cup of diced red bell pepper
- ¼ cup of minced red onion
- ½ cup of chopped spinach
- 1 tsp. of sea salt
- 1 tsp. of red chili powder
- 1/8 tsp. of Ground black pepper
- 1 cup of water
- 1 avocado (peeled, pitted, sliced)
- ½ cup of sour cream

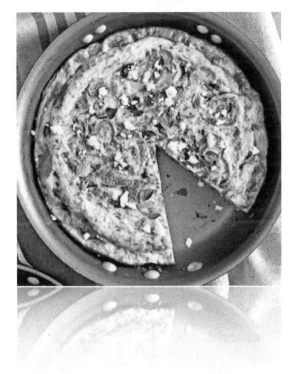

Kitchen Equipment:
- 7-inch baking dish
- instant pot
- trivet stand

Directions:

1. Break eggs in a bowl, add cream and whisk until beaten and fluffy.
2. Add remaining ingredients, except for water, avocado and sour cream, stir well until incorporated and then pour the mixture in a 7-inch baking dish greased with avocado oil.
3. Switch on the instant pot, pour water in it, insert a trivet stand and place baking dish on it.
4. Seal the instant pot, then click the 'manual' button, press '+/-' to adjust the cooking time to 12 minutes and press high-pressure setting; when the pressure starts, the timer will start.
5. When the instant pot rings, select the 'keep warm' button, let the pressure release naturally for 10 minutes. Then slowly open the pot.
6. Take out the baking dish and take out the frittata by inverting the dish onto a plate, and cut into slices.
7. Serve straight away.

Nutrition: Calories: 218 - **Fat:** 17.6g - **Protein:** 9.4g

1. Low Carb Gnocchi

Preparation Time: 20 minutes

Cooking Time: 15 minutes

Servings: 2

Ingredients:

- 3 egg yolks (large)
- ½ teaspoon of garlic powder
- 2 cups of mozzarella (low moisture, shredded, park skim)
- 1 teaspoon of salt

Kitchen Equipment:

- oven
- silicon spatula
- parchment paper
- pot

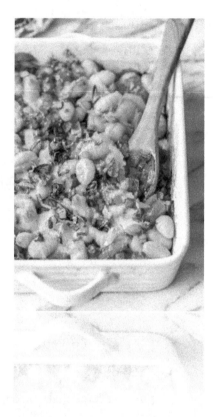

Directions:

1. Sprinkle mozzarella with the seasonings and then melt it in a toaster oven for 10 minutes, continue stirring it.

2. Split the egg yolks from whites and beat them until well mixed.

3. Combine the melted mozzarella with half of the egg yolks mixture using two silicone spatulas.

4. Once everything is well mixed, separate it into ¼; rolling each fourth into a thin and long strip on a parchment paper piece.

5. Cut approximately 1" pieces in every strip until you have plenty of cheese gnocchi.

6. To make them look like more traditional gnocchi; gently press a fork onto them.

7. Fill a pot with water and bring it to a boil, over moderate heat; carefully drop the pieces of gnocchi into the boiling water.

8. Boil them until starts floating and then drain.

9. The next step is to fry the gnocchi on an oiled pan on both sides.

10. Enjoy.

Nutrition: Calories: 440 - **Total Fat:** 32g - **Total Carbohydrates:** 3.9g

Easy Roasted Broccoli

Preparation Time: 2 minutes

Cooking Time: 19 minutes

Servings: 4

Ingredients:

- 1-pound of frozen broccoli (cut into florets)

- 3 tsp. of olive oil

- Sea salt (to taste)

Kitchen Equipment:

- baking sheet

- oven

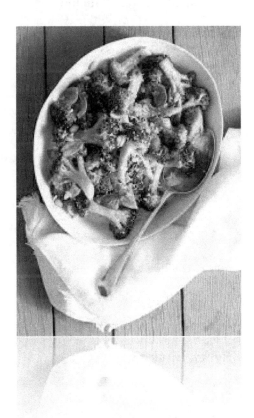

Directions:

1. Place broccoli florets on a baking sheet greased with oil and put it in the oven (preheated to 400°F).

2. Sprinkle the olive oil over the florets.

3. Cook for 12 minutes.

4. Whisk well and bake for additional 7 minutes.

Nutrition:

- **Fat:** 3g

- **Protein:** 3g

- **Calories:** 58

Chicken Pan with Veggies and Pesto

Preparation Time: 10 minutes

Cooking Time: 20 minutes

Servings: 4

Ingredients:

- 2 tbsp. of olive oil
- 1-pound of chicken thighs (boneless, skinless, sliced into strips)
- ¾ cup of oil-packed sun-dried tomatoes (chopped)
- 1-pound of asparagus ends
- ¼ cup of basil pesto
- 1 cup of cherry tomatoes (red and yellow, halved)
- Salt (to taste)

Kitchen Equipment:

- frying pan
- skillet

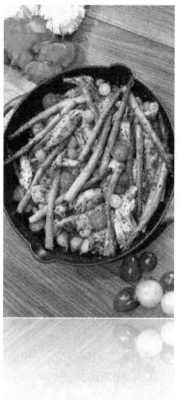

Directions:

1. Cook olive oil in a frying pan over medium-high heat.
2. Put salt on the chicken slices and then put into a skillet, add the sun-dried tomatoes and fry for 5–10 minutes.
3. Remove the chicken slices and season with salt.
4. Add asparagus to the skillet.
5. Cook for additional 5–10 minutes.
6. Transfer the chicken back in the skillet, pour in the pesto and whisk.
7. Fry for 1–2 minutes.
8. Remove from the heat.
9. Add the halved cherry tomatoes and pesto.
10. Stir well and serve.

Nutrition: Carbohydrates: 12g - **Protein:** 2g - **Calories:** 423

Turkey-Pepper Mix

Preparation Time: 20 minutes

Cooking Time: 0 minute

Servings: 1

Ingredients:

- 1-pound of turkey tenderloin (cut in thin steaks)

- 1 tsp. of salt, divided)

- 2 tbsp. of extra-virgin olive oil (divided)

- ½ sweet onion (sliced)

- 1 red bell pepper (cut into strips)

- 1 yellow bell pepper (cut into strips)

- ½ tsp. of Italian seasoning

- ¼ tsp. of ground black pepper

- 2 tsp. of red wine vinegar

- 1 14-ounces can of crushed tomatoes, roasted

- Fresh parsley

- Basil

Kitchen Equipment:

- pan

Directions:

1. Sprinkle ½ tsp. of salt on your turkey.

2. Drizzle 1 tablespoon of oil into the pan and heat it.

3. Add the turkey steaks and cook for 1–3 minutes per side. Set aside.

4. Put the onion, bell peppers, and the remaining salt to the pan and cook for 7 minutes, stirring all the time.

5. Sprinkle with Italian seasoning and add black pepper.

6. Cook for 30 seconds.

7. Add the tomatoes and vinegar and fry the mix for about 20 seconds.

8. Place the turkey back to the pan and pour the sauce over it.

9. Simmer for 2–3 minutes.

10. Top with chopped parsley and basil.

Nutrition:

- **Carbohydrates:** 11g

- **Protein:** 30g

- **Calories:** 230

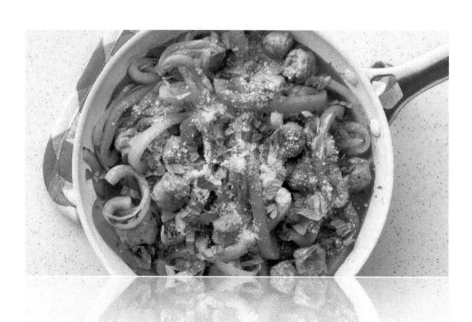

Tuscan Truffles

Preparation Time: 10 minutes

Cooking Time: 25 minutes

Servings: 6

Ingredients:

- 2 logs of goat cheese
- 8 ounces of mascarpone cheese
- 6 tbsps. of parmesan cheese (grated)
- 3 cloves of garlic (minced)
- 2 tsps. of olive oil
- 1 tsp. of white balsamic vinegar
- 3/4 tsp. of lemon zest (grated)
- 6 ½ tbsp. of prosciutto (chopped)
- 5 tbsps. of dried figs (chopped)
- 3 tbsps. of parsley (minced)
- ¼ tsp. of pepper
- 1 cup of pine nuts (chopped)

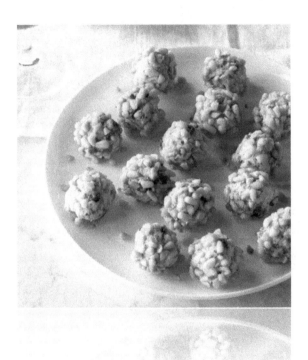

Kitchen Equipment:

- large bowl

Directions:

1. Mix the first eleven listed ingredients in a large bowl.

2. Shape the mixture into thirty-six small balls.

3. Roll the balls in chopped pine nuts.

4. Refrigerate for twenty minutes.

Nutrition: Calories: 82.3 - **Protein:** 3.3g - **Fat:** 7.3g

Caprese Salad Kabobs

Preparation Time: 10 minutes

Cooking Time: 10 minutes

Servings: 4 servings

Ingredients:

- 24 grape tomatoes

- 12 small bits of mozzarella cheese balls

- 24 basil leaves

- 3 tbsps. of olive oil

- 2 tsps. of balsamic vinegar

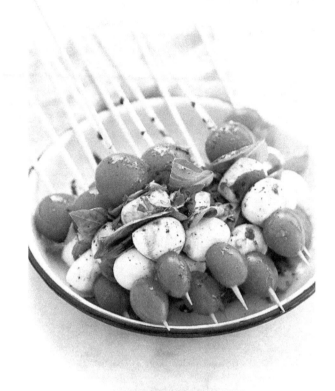

Kitchen Equipment:

- small bowl

- skewers

Directions:

1. Combine vinegar along with olive oil in a small bowl.

2. Thread two tomatoes, two leaves of basil, and one ball of cheese alternately on each skewer.

3. Drizzle the mixture of olive oil over the skewers.

4. Serve immediately.

Nutrition:

- **Calories:** 45.4

- **Protein:** 2.3g - **Carbs:** 1.6g

Zucchini Crusted Pizza

Preparation Time: 10 minutes

Cooking Time: 45 minutes

Servings: 6

Ingredients:

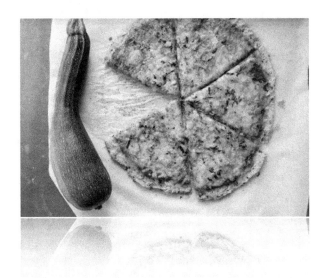

- 2 large eggs (beaten)
- 2 cups of zucchini (shredded, squeezed)
- ½ cup of mozzarella cheese (shredded)
- 1/3 cup of parmesan cheese (grated)
- ¼ cup of flour
- 1 tbsp. of olive oil
- 1 ½ tbsp. of basil (minced)
- 1 tsp. of thyme (minced)

For the toppings:

- 12 ounces of sweet red pepper (roasted, julienned)
- 1 cup of mozzarella cheese (shredded)
- ½ cup of turkey pepperoni (sliced)

Kitchen Equipment:

- oven
- pizza pan
- pizza cutter

Directions:

1. Preheat your oven at two hundred degrees Celsius.
2. Mix the first eight listed ingredients in a bowl.
3. Transfer the mixture to a greased pizza pan.
4. Spread the mixture and evenly press it to the base.
5. Bake for sixteen minutes.
6. Add the toppings on the pizza.
7. Bake for twelve minutes.
8. Slice the pizza using a pizza cutter.
9. Serve hot.

Nutrition:

- **Calories:** 226.3 - **Protein:** 13.6g - **Carbs:** 8.6g

Mushroom and Asparagus Frittata

Preparation Time: 10 minutes

Cooking Time: 45 minutes

Servings: 8

Ingredients:

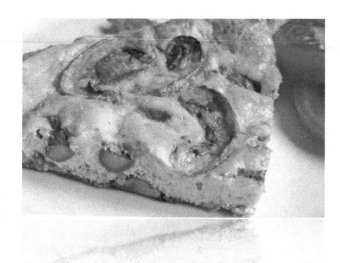

- 8 large eggs
- 1/2 cup of ricotta cheese
- 2 tbsps. of lemon juice
- 1/2 tsp. of salt
- 1/4 tsp. of pepper
- 1 tbsp. of olive oil
- 8 ounces of asparagus spears
- 1 onion (sliced)
- 1/3 cup of sweet green pepper
- 3/4 cup of Portobello mushrooms (sliced)

Kitchen Equipment:

- oven
- iron skillet

Directions:

1. Preheat your oven at one hundred and fifty degrees Celsius.
2. Mix ricotta cheese, eggs, pepper, lemon juice, and salt in a bowl.
3. Heat oil in an iron skillet.
4. Add onion, asparagus, mushrooms, and red pepper.
5. Cook for eight minutes.
6. Remove the asparagus from the skillet.
7. Cut the spears of asparagus into pieces of 2-inch.
8. Return the spears to the skillet.
9. Add the mixture of eggs.
10. Bake in the oven for twenty minutes.
11. Let the frittata sit for five minutes.
12. Cut the frittata into wedges. Serve warm.

Nutrition:

- **Calories:** 132.2 - **Protein:** 9.3g - **Fat:** 8.2g

Frittata

Preparation Time: 5 minutes

Cooking Time: 17 minutes

Servings: 1

Ingredients:

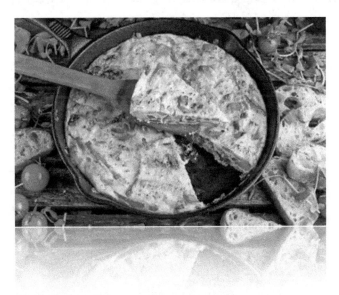

- 5oz of bacon slices (pastured, diced)
- ½ medium red onion (peeled, diced)
- ½ red bell pepper (cored, diced)
- ¼ tsp. of salt
- 1 tsp. of ground black pepper
- 3 tbsp. of avocado oil
- ¼ cup and 2 tbsp. of grated parmesan cheese (full-fat)
- 6 eggs (pastured)

Kitchen Equipment:

- 8-inch skillet pan
- broiler
- microwave

Directions:

1. Take an 8-inches skillet pan, grease with oil and place it over medium heat.
2. Add onion, pepper and bacon, cook for 5 minutes or until slightly golden and then season with salt and black pepper.
3. Beat the eggs in a bowl, add ¼ cup of cheese and whisk until mixed.
4. When bacon is cooked, pour the egg mixture into the pan, spread evenly and cook for 5 minutes or until frittata is set.
5. In the meantime, switch on the broiler and let preheat.
6. When the frittata is set, sprinkle remaining cheese on the top, then place the pan under the broiler and cook until golden brown.
7. Let the frittata cool at room temperature, then cut it into four pieces, place each frittata piece in a heatproof glass meal prep container and store them in the refrigerator for 5 to 7 days.
8. When ready to serve, microwave frittata in their container for 1 to 2 minutes or until thoroughly heated.

Nutrition: Calories: 494 - **Fat:** 40g - **Protein:** 32g

Stuffed Eggs with Bacon-Avocado Filling

Preparation Time: 10 minutes

Cooking Time: 10 minutes

Servings: 1

Ingredients:

- 2 eggs (boiled and halved)

- 1 tbsp. of mayonnaise

- ¼ tsp. of mustard

- 1/8 lemon (squeezed)

- ¼ tsp. of garlic powder

- 1/8 tsp. of salt

- 1/8 tsp. of smoked paprika

- ¼ avocado

- 16 small pieces of bacon

Kitchen Equipment:

- frying pan

Directions:

1. Fry the bacon for 3 minutes in a pan.

2. Add the avocado and fry for additional 3 minutes (lower heat).

3. Combine the mayonnaise, mustard, lemon, garlic powder, and salt in a separate bowl.

4. Stir well.

5. Take out the yolk from the halved eggs and fill the egg halves with the mayonnaise mix.

6. Top with the bacon-avocado filling.

Nutrition:

- **Carbohydrates:** 14g

- **Fat:** 30g

- **Calories:** 342

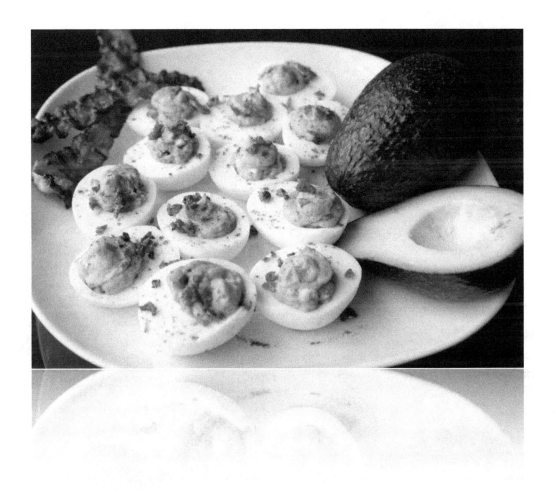

Balsamic Chicken

Preparation Time: 10 minutes

Cooking Time: 60 minutes

Servings: 4

Ingredients:

- 4 pcs. of chicken breast

- 2 tbsp. of grass-fed butter

- A dash salt

- 4 roasted garlic cloves

- 2 cups of mushrooms

- 1 tsp. of thyme

- 1 tbsp. of chives

- 1 tsp. of red pepper flakes

- ¼ cup of balsamic vinegar

- ½ cup of water

- ¼ cup of onions

Kitchen Equipment:

- stove

- baking sheet

- skillet

Directions:

1. Prepare the stove to 350 and getting out your baking sheet.

2. As the stove warms up, take out your skillet and begin heating the butter in it. Once melted, mix in the chicken pieces and season with your pepper and salt. When the meat is seasoned to your taste, grill each side of the chicken for 3 or 4 minutes. Once it's cooked thoroughly, transfer it onto your baking sheet, and cook in your heated stove for additional 25 minutes.

3. While the chicken cooks, melt some more butter in your heated pan. Once melted, sauté mushrooms and onions. Mix in the roasted garlic, thyme, red pepper flakes, and the balsamic vinegar. After these ingredients have cooked for a minute, pour in the water and stir until the liquid begins to reduce.

4. Pour the mixture over your chicken and serve the dish hot. If you would like, you can serve with fresh parsley or chopped chives for some nice additional flavors.

Nutrition:

Fats: 15g

Carbs: 8g

Proteins: 30g

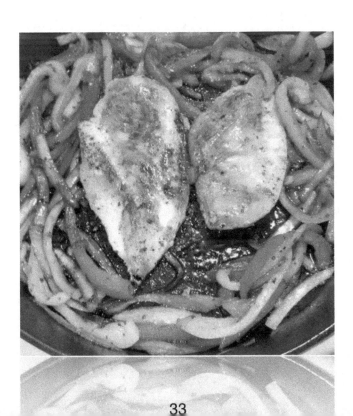

Cheesy Keto Meatballs

Preparation Time: 15 minutes

Cooking Time: 20 minutes

Servings: 3

Ingredients:

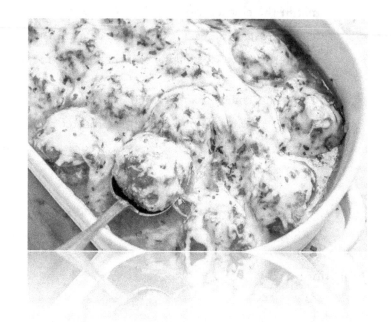

- 1 lb. of ground beef

- A dash of salt

- 1 tsp. of garlic powder

- 3 tbsp. of parmesan cheese

- 1 cup of mozzarella cheese

- A dash of pepper

Kitchen Equipment:

- frying pan

Directions:

1. Chop your fresh mozzarella into bite-sized pieces.

2. Season the ground beef to your taste and then carefully wrap each cheese piece with the ground beef and begin creating your meatballs.

3. Once you are set to cook your meal, take out your frying pan and place it over a moderate temperature. When the pan is warm, you can go ahead and grill the meatballs on all sides for 5 minutes or so. By the end of this time, the meatballs should be crispy and can be served over some zoodles or enjoyed by themselves!

Nutrition: Fats: 35g - **Carbs:** 2g - **Proteins:** 40g

Lasagna Stuffed Peppers

Preparation Time: 15 minutes

Cooking Time: 1 hour and 5 minutes

Servings: 6

Ingredients:

- 6 large bell pepper (destemmed, cored)

- 1 ½ lb. of ground beef (pastured)

- 2 tbsp. of minced garlic

- ¾ tsp. of sea salt

- ½ tsp. of ground black pepper

- 2 cups of marinara sauce (organic)

- 1 tbsp. of Italian seasoning

- 1 cup of ricotta cheese (full-fat)

- 1 cup of mozzarella cheese (full-fat, shredded)

Kitchen Equipment:

- skillet pan

- oven

- baking sheet

- aluminum foil

Directions:

1. Prepare the meat sauce and for this, place a skillet pan over medium-high heat, grease with oil, then add garlic and cook for 30 seconds until fragrant.

2. Then add beef, stir well, cook for 10 minutes until nicely browned, season with salt, black pepper and marinara sauce, stir well and simmer the sauce for 10 minutes.

3. Meanwhile, set an oven to 375 degrees F and let preheat.

4. When the meat sauce is cooked, remove the pan from the oven and let cool for 5 minutes.

5. In the meantime, prepare the peppers and for this, cut off the tops, then scoop the inside seeds and ribs and slice slightly from the bottoms, without making any holes, so that peppers can stand upright.

6. Assemble the peppers and for this, spoon 2 tablespoons of prepared meat sauce in the bottom of peppers, then evenly top with ricotta cheese and mozzarella cheese, and add two more layers in the same manner with mozzarella cheese on the top.

7. Take a baking sheet, line it with aluminum foil, place the stuffed peppers on it and then tent with aluminum foil.

8. Situate the baking sheet into the oven, bake for 30 minutes, then remove the aluminum foil and continue baking for 10 minutes or until cheese melts and slightly browned.

9. Cool the stuffed pepper at room temperature, then wrap each pepper with aluminum foil and store in the freezer for about 2 to 3 minutes.

10. When ready to serve, reheat the peppers into the oven at 350 degrees F for 5 minutes or until hot.

Nutrition:

Calories: 412

Fat: 27g

Protein: 30g

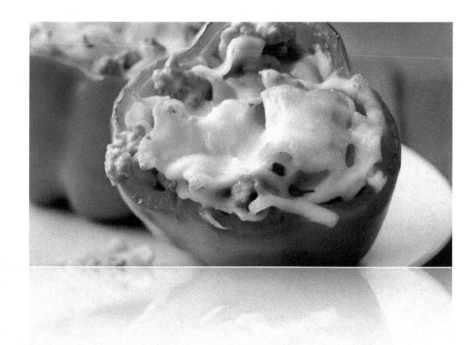

Cold Avocado and Crab Soup

Preparation Time: 15 minutes

Cooking Time: 0 minute

Servings: 6

Ingredients:

- ½ onion, diced

- ½ cup of fresh cilantro, roughly chopped

- 1 cup of watercress

- 1 cup of heavy whipping cream

- 1 English cucumber, cut into chunks

- 2 avocados, diced

- 2 cups of coconut water

- 2 teaspoons of ground cumin

- Juice of 1 lime

- Salt and black pepper, to taste

- 1 pound (454 g) of cooked crab meat

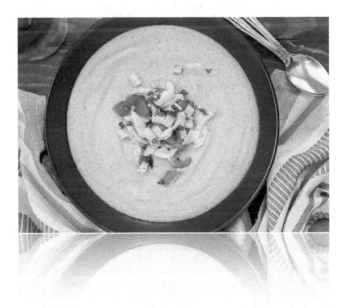

Kitchen Equipment:

- blender

- large bowl

Directions:

1. Incorporate all the ingredients, except for the crab meat, in a blender.

2. Process until smooth.

3. Pour the soup in a large bowl.

4. Add the crab meat into the soup and serve immediately

Nutrition: Calories: 298 - **Total fat:** 23.1g - **Fiber:** 4.1g

Sautéed Crispy Zucchini

Gluten Free, Nut Free, Vegetarian

Preparation Time: 15 minutes

Cooking Time: 10 minutes

Servings: 4

Ingredients:

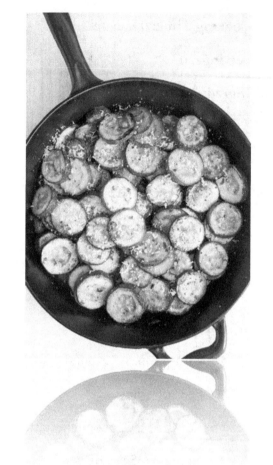

- 2 tablespoons of butter

- 4 zucchinis, cut into ¼-inch-thick rounds

- ½ cup of freshly grated Parmesan cheese

- Freshly ground black pepper

Kitchen Equipment:

- large skillet

Directions:

1. Cook butter over medium-high heat in a large skillet.

2. Stir in the zucchini and sauté until tender and lightly browned, about 5 minutes.

3. Arrange the zucchini evenly in the skillet and topped it with Parmesan cheese over the vegetables.

4. Continue cooking it without stirring until the Parmesan cheese is melted and crispy where it touches the skillet, about 5 minutes.

5. Serve.

Nutrition: Calories: 94 - **Fat:** 8g - **Protein:** 4g

Pesto Zucchini Noodles

Gluten Free, Nut Free, Vegetarian

Preparation Time: 15 minutes

Cooking Time: 15 minutes

Servings: 4

Ingredients:

- 4 small zucchinis, ends trimmed

- ¾ cup Herb Kale Pesto

- ¼ cup grated or shredded

- Parmesan cheese

Kitchen Equipment:

- spiralizer or peeler

- medium bowl

Directions:

1. Make the zucchini into noodles by using a spiralizer and place them in a medium bowl.

2. Add the pesto and the Parmesan cheese and toss to coat.

3. Serve.

Nutrition:

Calories: 93

Fat: 8g

Protein: 4g

Crispy Parmesan Crackers

Gluten Free, Nut Free, Vegetarian

Preparation Time: 10 minutes

Cooking Time: 5 minutes

Servings: 8

Ingredients:

- 1 teaspoon of butter

- 8 ounces of full-fat Parmesan cheese, shredded or freshly grated

Kitchen Equipment:

- oven

- baking sheet

- parchment paper

- spatula

- container

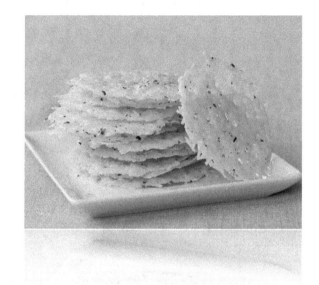

Directions:

1. Preheat the oven to 400 degrees.

2. Put parchment paper in a baking sheet and lightly grease the paper with the butter.

3. Spoon the Parmesan cheese onto the baking sheet in mounds, spread evenly apart.

4. Spread out the mounds with the back of a spoon until they are flat.

5. Bake the crackers until the edges are browned and the centers are still pale, about 5 minutes.

6. Pull out the sheet from the oven, and remove the crackers with a spatula to paper towels.

7. Lightly blot the tops with additional paper towels and let them completely cool.

8. Store in a sealed container in the refrigerator for up to 4 days.

Nutrition: Calories: 133 - **Fat:** 11g - **Protein:** 11g

8 Ingredient Zucchini Lasagna

Preparation Time: 10 minutes

Cooking Time: 1 hour 20 minutes

Servings: 9

Ingredients:

For ricotta:

- 3 cups of raw macadamia nuts

- 2 tbsp. of nutritional yeast

- 2 tsp. of dried oregano

- 1 tsp. of sea salt

- 1/2 cup of water

- 1/4 cup of vegan parmesan cheese

- 1/2 cup of fresh basil, chopped

- 1 medium lemon, juiced

- Black pepper to taste

Sauce:

- 1 28-oz jar favorite marinara sauce

- 3 medium zucchini squash thinly sliced

Kitchen Equipment:

- mandolin

- oven

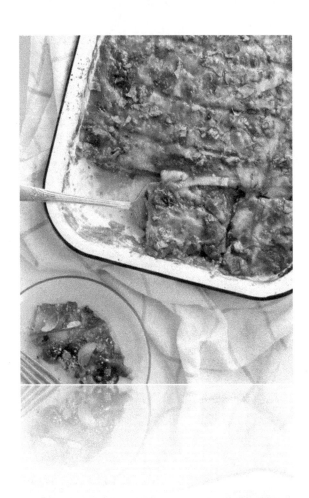

- food processor

- pan

- aluminum foil

Directions:

1. Prepare the oven to 375 degrees Fahrenheit.

2. Put macadamia nuts to a food processor.

3. Add the remaining ingredients and continue to puree the mixture. You need to create a fine paste.

4. Taste and adjust the seasonings depending on your personal preferences.

5. Pour 1 cup of marinara sauce in a baking dish.

6. Start creating the lasagna layers using thinly sliced zucchini

7. Scoop small amounts of ricotta mixture on the zucchini and spread it into a thin layer.

8. Continue the layering until you've run out of zucchini or space for it.

9. Sprinkle parmesan cheese on the topmost layer.

10. Wrap it with foil then bake for 45 minutes.

11. Remove the foil and bake for 15 minutes more.

12. Allow it to cool for 15 minutes before serving.

13. Serve immediately.

14. The lasagna will keep for 3 days in the fridge.

Nutrition:

Calories: 338

Fat: 34g

Carbohydrates: 10g

No-Churn Ice Cream

Preparation Time: 10 minutes plus 80 minutes chilling time

Cooking Time: 0 minute

Servings: 3

Ingredients:

- Pinch salt

- 1 cup of heavy whipping cream

- ¼ tsp. of xanthan gum

- 2 tbsp. of zero calorie sweetener powder

- 1 tsp. of vanilla extract

- 1 tbsp. of vodka

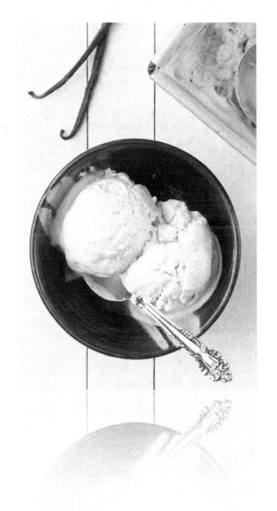

Kitchen Equipment:

- immersion blender

- wide-mouth jar

Directions:

1. You'll need an immersion blender and a jar that is pint sized with a wide mouth. First, add the xanthan gum, heavy cream, vanilla extract, sweetener, vodka, and salt to a jar and mix.

2. Transfer the mixture to the immersion blender and, with the up-down motion, blend until you are left with a thick mixture. This should take up to 2 minutes.

3. Put the mixture back in the jar, cover it, and place it in your freezer for 4 hours. Remember to stir the cream mixture in 40 minutes intervals.

Nutrition: Calories: 291 - **Protein:** 1.6g - **Fat:** 29.4g

Strawberries with Coconut Whip

Preparation Time: 10 minutes

Cooking Time: 0 minute

Servings: 4

Ingredients:

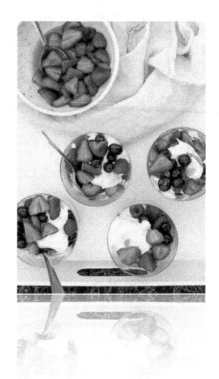

- 4 cups of strawberries or other favorite berries

- 2 cans of refrigerated coconut cream

- 1 oz. 70% or darker unsweetened chopped dark chocolate

Kitchen Equipment:

- hand mixer

Directions:

1. Remove the solidified cream from the can of milk and set aside for another time, saving the liquid.

2. Pour it into a mixing container and whip with a hand mixer until it forms stiff peaks (approximately five minutes).

3. Slice the berries and divide into four dishes.

4. Serve with a dollop of the cream.

5. Garnish with the chopped chocolate and a few berries.

6. Serve.

Nutrition:

Net Carbohydrates: 10g

Protein: 4g

Calories: 342

Hot Chocolate Ice Cream

Preparation Time: 45 minutes

Cooking Time: 0 minute

Servings: 12

Ingredients:

- 2 cans of chilled coconut milk

- 1-4 scoops chocolate protein powder

- 2 tbsp. of cocoa powder

- 2 tbsp. of granulated sweetener (ex. Monk fruit)

Kitchen Equipment:

- 1 deep loaf pan

- food processor or blender

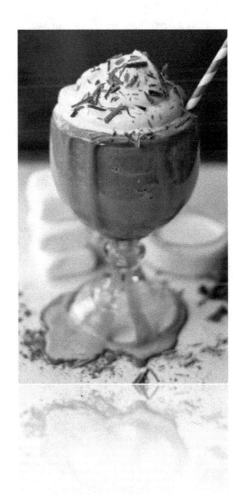

Directions:

1. Situate the pan in the freezer to chill.

2. Take the can of milk out of the fridge and split the water from the cream.

3. Add the cream into a food processor or high-speed blender, followed by the coconut water.

4. Blend until just combined.

5. Add the protein powder, granulated sweetener, and cocoa powder.

6. Blend until it's thick and creamy, but don't over-blend.

7. Add the ice cream to the chilled pan. Lightly stir the ice cream every 20–30 minutes for the first hour to help prevent it from becoming too icy. When it's time to serve, thaw the loaf pan for approximately 15 minutes.

Nutrition:

Protein: 7g **Total - Fats:** 11g - **Calories:** 130

Raspberry Soft-Serve Ice Cream

Preparation Time: 60 minutes

Cooking Time: 0 minute

Servings: 5

Ingredients:

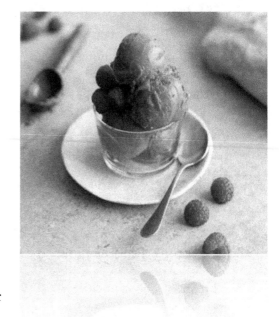

- 1 cup of heavy cream or coconut cream

- 2 cups of frozen raspberries

- 1/3 cup of powdered erythritol or any sweetener

Kitchen Equipment:

- blender or hand mixer

Directions:

1. Pour the cream into a blender.

2. Blend until stiff peaks form (You can also use a hand mixer if your blender isn't powerful enough to whip the cream).

3. Toss the frozen raspberries and sweetener into the blender. Puree until incorporated.

4. Adjust the sweetener to taste if needed, and if added, puree again.

5. For firmer ice cream, run the mixture through an ice cream maker, or place in the freezer to firm up.

6. Stir every 30–60 minutes for the first couple hours to break up any ice crystals.

Nutrition:

Protein: 1g

Total Fats: 16g

Calories: 183

Avocado Egg Bake

Preparation Time: 5 minutes

Cooking Time: 15 minutes

Servings: 1

Ingredients:

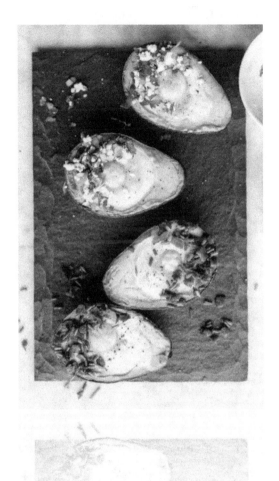

- 1 tbsp. of fresh parsley, chopped

- 1 avocado, cut in half and the pits removed

- Salt to taste

- Ground black pepper to your preferred taste

- 2 eggs

- ¼ cup of cheddar cheese shredded

Kitchen Equipment:

- oven

- baking sheet

Directions:

1. Preheat the oven to 425 degrees F.

2. The next thing to do is scoop some avocado from the pitted area.

3. Place both halves of the avocado on a baking sheet and break an egg onto each avocado.

4. Let it bake in the oven for about 20 minutes. Only stop baking when you are sure the eggs are cooked.

5. Add salt and pepper to season the avocado egg, and garnish with cheddar cheese and parsley.

Nutrition: Calories: 605 - **Protein:** 25.3g - **Fat:** 50.9g

Lemon Cheesecake

Preparation Time: 10 minutes

Cooking Time: 55 minutes

Servings: 8

Ingredients:

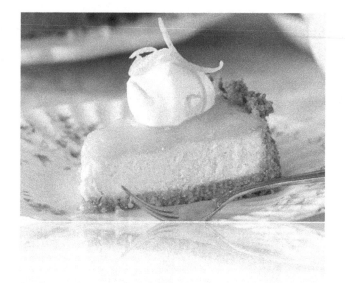

- 4 eggs

- 18 oz. of ricotta cheese

- 1 fresh lemon zest

- 2 tbsp. of swerve

- 1 fresh lemon juice

Kitchen Equipment:

- oven

- cake pan

Directions:

1. Prepare oven at 350 F/ 180C.

2. Spray cake pan with cooking spray then set aside.

3. Beat ricotta cheese until smooth.

4. Add egg one by one and whisk well.

5. Add lemon juice, lemon zest, and swerve and mix well.

6. Transfer mixture into the prepared cake pan and bake for 50–55 minutes.

7. Pull out the cake from oven and set aside to cool completely.

8. Place cake in the fridge for 1–2 hours.

9. Slice and serve.

Nutrition:

Calories: 12 - **Total Fat:** 7.3g - **Protein:** 10.2g

Chapter 4. Recipes from Greece

Chocolate Protein Pancakes

Preparation Time: 10 minutes

Cooking Time: 15 minutes

Servings: 12

Ingredients:

- ½ cup of almond flour, blanched

- ½ cup of whey protein powder

- 1 tsp. of baking powder

- 1/8 tsp. of sea salt

- 3 tbsp. of erythritol sweetener

- 1 tsp. of vanilla extract, unsweetened

- 3 tbsp. of cocoa powder, organic, unsweetened

- 4 Eggs, pastured

- 2 tbsp. of avocado oil

- 1/3 cup of almond milk, unsweetened

Kitchen Equipment:

- immersion blender

- medium skillet pan

- freezer bag

- parchment paper

- microwave or oven

Directions:

1. Transfer all the ingredients in a large mixing bowl, beat using an immersion blender or until well combined and then let the mixture stand for 5 minutes.

2. Then take a medium skillet pan, place it over medium-low heat, grease it with avocado oil and pour in prepared pancake batter in small circles of about 3-inches diameter.

3. Cover the skillet pan with lid, let the pancakes cook for 3 minutes or until bubbles form on top, then flip them and continue cooking for 1 to 2 minutes or until nicely golden brown.

4. Cook remaining pancakes, in the same manner, you will end up with 12 pancakes, and then let them cool at room temperature.

5. Place cooled pancakes in a freezer bag, with parchment sheet between them and store them in the refrigerator for 5 to 7 days.

6. When ready to serve, microwave pancakes for 30 seconds to 1 minute or bake in the oven for 5 minutes until thoroughly heated.

Nutrition:

Calories: 237

Fat: 20g

Protein: 11g

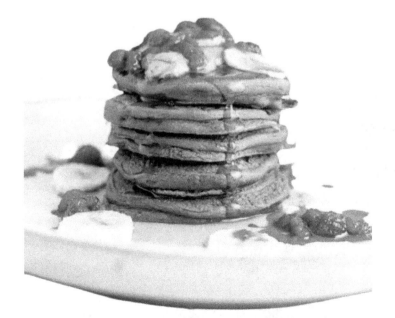

Blueberry Pancake Bites

Preparation Time: 10 minutes

Cooking Time: 25 minutes

Servings: 24

Ingredients:

- ½ cup of frozen blueberries

- ½ cup of coconut flour

- 1 tsp. of baking powder

- ½ tsp. of salt

- ¼ cup of swerve Sweetener

- ¼ tsp. of cinnamon

- ½ tsp. of vanilla extract, unsweetened

- ¼ cup of butter, grass-fed, unsalted, melted

- 4 Eggs, pastured

- 1/3 cup of water

Kitchen Equipment:

- oven

- immersion blender

- silicon mini muffin tray

- freezer bag

Directions:

1. Prepare oven at 350 degrees.

2. Crack the eggs in a bowl, add vanilla and sweetener, whisk using an immersion blender until blended and then blend in salt, cinnamon, butter, baking powder, and flour until incorporated and smooth batter comes together.

3. Let the batter rest until thickened and then blend in water until combined.

4. Take a 25-cups silicone mini-muffin tray, grease the cups with avocado oil, then evenly scoop the prepared batter in them and top with few blueberries, pressing the berries gently into the batter.

5. Situate the muffin tray into the oven and bake the muffins for 25 minutes or until thoroughly cooked and the top is nicely golden brown.

6. When done, take out muffins from the tray and cool them on the wire rack.

7. Place muffins in a large freezer bag or evenly divide them in packets and store them in the refrigerator for four days.

8. When ready to serve, microwave the muffins for 45 seconds to 1 minute or until thoroughly heated.

Nutrition:

Calories: 188

Fat: 13.8g

Protein: 5.7g

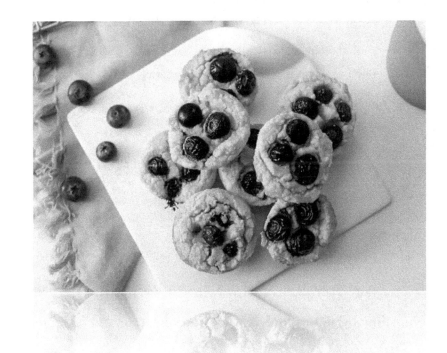

Almond Flour Keto Pancakes

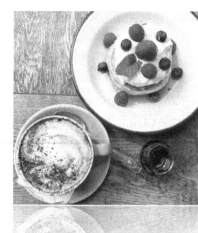

Preparation Time: 10 minutes

Cooking Time: 12 minutes

Servings: 10

Ingredients:

- 4 oz. of softened cream cheese, at room temperature

- Zest of 1 medium-sized lemon, fresh (approximately 1 teaspoon)

- 4 large-sized eggs, organic

- ½ cup of almond flour

- 1 tablespoon of butter, for frying and serving

Kitchen Equipment:

- medium-size mixing bowl

- nonstick skillet

Directions:

1. Combine the almond flour with eggs, cream cheese, and lemon zest using a whisk in a medium-sized mixing bowl until combined well, and completely smooth, for a minute or two.

2. The next step is to heat a large, nonstick skillet over medium heat until hot.

3. Once done, add 1 tablespoon of butter until completely melted; swirl to coat the bottom completely.

4. Pour 3 tablespoons of the prepared batter (for each pancake) and cook for a minute or two, until turn golden.

5. Carefully flip, cook the other side for 2 more minutes.

6. Transfer to a clean, large plate and continue cooking with the remaining batter.

7. Top the cooked pancakes with some butter; serve immediately and enjoy.

Nutrition: Calories: 120 - **Total Carbohydrates:** 2g - **Protein:** 3.9g

Baked Carrot with Bacon

Preparation Time: 10 minutes

Cooking Time: 35 minutes

Servings: 4

Ingredients:

- 1½ pounds of carrot, peeled

- 12 slices bacon

- 1 tbsp. of black pepper

- 1/3 cup of maple syrup

- 1 pinch parsley

Kitchen Equipment:

- oven

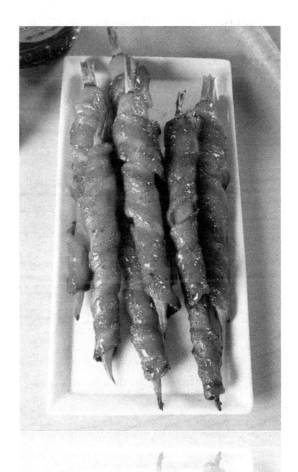

Directions:

1. Preheat the oven to 400°F.

2. Wrap the bacon slices around your carrots from top to bottom, add black pepper, sprinkle with maple syrup and bake for about 20–25 minutes.

3. Top with parsley and serve.

Nutrition:

Fat: 26g

Protein: 10g

Calories: 421

Roasted Cauliflower and Tahini Yogurt Sauce

Preparation Time: 10 minutes

Cooking Time: 55 minutes

Servings: 4

Ingredients:

- ¼ cup of parmesan cheese (grated)

- 3 tbsps. of olive oil

- 2 cloves of garlic (minced)

- ¼ tsp. of salt

- 1/3 tsp. of pepper

- 1 cauliflower (cut in four wedges)

For the sauce:

- ½ cup of Greek yogurt

- 1 tbsp. of lemon juice

- ½ tbsp. of tahini

- ¼ tsp. of salt

- 1 pinch of paprika

- Parsley (minced)

Kitchen Equipment:

- oven

- baking tray

Directions:

1. Preheat your oven at one hundred and fifty degrees Celsius.

2. Mix the first five ingredients.

3. Rub the mixture over the wedges of cauliflower.

4. Grease a baking tray with cooking spray.

5. Arrange the wedges of cauliflower on the baking tray.

6. Roast for forty minutes.

7. For the sauce, combine lemon juice, yogurt, seasonings, and tahini in a bowl.

8. Serve the cauliflower wedges and drizzle tahini sauce on top.

9. Garnish with parsley.

Nutrition:

Calories: 179.6

Protein: 7.6g

Fat: 15.4g

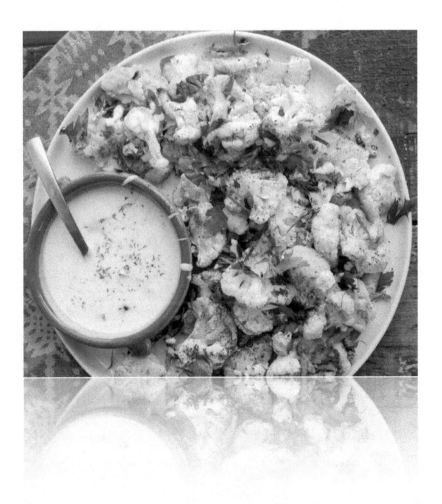

Cobb Salad Sausage Lettuce Wraps

Preparation Time: 10 minutes

Cooking Time: 25 minutes

Servings: 6

Ingredients:

- 3/4 cup of ranch salad dressing
- 1/3 cup of blue cheese (crumbled)
- 1/4 cup of watercress (chopped)
- 1 pound of pork sausage
- 2 tbsps. of chives (minced)
- 6 leaves of iceberg lettuce
- 1 avocado (peeled, diced)
- 4 boiled eggs (chopped)
- 1 tomato (chopped)

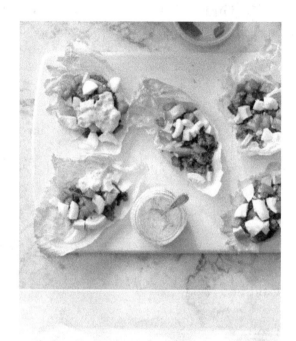

Kitchen Equipment:

- iron skillet

Directions:

1. Combine blue cheese, dressing, and watercress in a bowl.
2. Heat some oil in an iron skillet.
3. Add the sausage.
4. Cook for seven minutes and crumble.
5. Add the chives.
6. Spoon the sausage mixture into the leaves of lettuce.
7. Top the sausage mixture with eggs, tomato, and avocado.
8. Drizzle the mixture of dressing on top.
9. Serve immediately.

Nutrition: Calories: 430.6 - **Protein:** 16.5g - **Fat:** 39.6g

Ranch Cauliflower Crackers

Preparation Time: 10 minutes

Cooking Time: 70 minutes

Servings: 6

Ingredients:

- 12 ounces of cauliflower rice

- Cheesecloth

- 1 large egg

- 1 tbsp. of ranch salad dressing mix (dry)

- 1/8 tsp. of cayenne pepper

- 1 cup of parmesan cheese (shredded)

Kitchen Equipment:

- microwave

- strainer

- oven

- parchment paper

- baking tray

Directions:

1. Add the cauliflower rice in a large bowl.

2. Microwave for four minutes covered.

3. Transfer the cauliflower rice to a strainer lined with cheesecloth.

4. Squeeze out excess moisture.

5. Preheat oven at two hundred degrees Celsius.

6. Use parchment paper for lining a baking tray.

7. Combine egg, cauliflower rice, ranch mix, and pepper in a bowl.

8. Add the cheese.

9. Mix well.

10. Take two tbsps. of the mixture and stir in to the baking tray.

11. Flatten with your hands. The thinner you can make the mixture, the crispier will be the crackers.

12. Bake for ten minutes.

13. Flip the crackers.

14. Bake for ten minutes.

15. Serve warm.

Nutrition:

Calories: 29.6

Protein: 2.6g

Fat: 2.6g

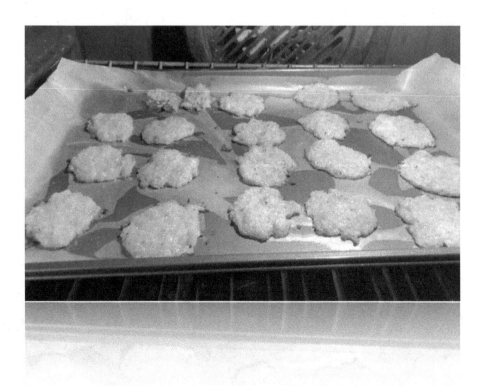

Roasted Cabbage with Bacon

Preparation Time: 10 minutes

Cooking Time: 40 minutes

Servings: 4

Ingredients:

- ½ head cabbage, quartered

- 8 slices bacon, cut into thick pieces

- ¼ cup of Parmesan cheese, grated

- 1 tsp. of garlic powder

- Salt and pepper, to taste

- 1 pinch parsley, chopped

Kitchen Equipment:

- baking sheet

- oven

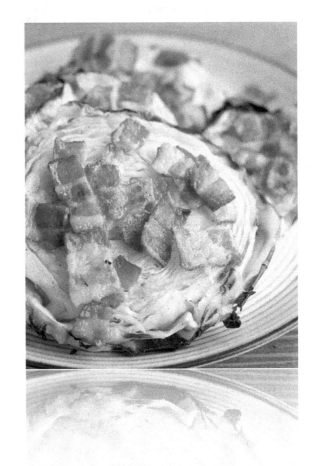

Directions:

1. Lightly sprinkle the cabbage wedges with the garlic powder and parmesan cheese.

2. Wrap 2 pieces of bacon around each cabbage wedge.

3. Place your wrapped cabbage wedges on the baking sheet and put into the oven preheated to 350°F oven.

4. Bake for 35–40 minutes.

5. Top with parsley.

Nutrition: Fat: 19g - **Protein:** 9g - **Calories:** 236

Spicy Tuna Kebabs

Preparation Time: 4 minutes

Cooking Time: 9 minutes

Servings: 4

Ingredients:

- 4 tablespoon of Huy Fong chili garlic sauce

- 1 tablespoon of sesame oil infused with garlic

- 1 tablespoon of ginger, fresh, grated

- 1 tablespoon of garlic, minced

- 1 red onion, separated by petals

- 2 cups of bell peppers, red, green, yellow

- 1 can of whole water chestnuts

- ½ pound of fresh mushrooms halved

- 32 oz. of boneless tuna, chunks or steaks

- 1 Splenda packet

- 2 zucchinis, sliced

- 1 inch thick, keep skins on

Kitchen Equipment:

- blender

- zip-lock bag

Directions:

1. Layer the tuna spices and the oil and chili gravy, add the Splenda.

2. Quickly blend, either in a blender or by quickly whipping.

3. Brush onto the kabob pieces, make sure every piece is coated

4. Grill 4 minutes on each district, check to ensure the tuna is cooked to taste. Serving size is two skewers.

5. Mix the marinade ingredients and hide in a covered container in the fridge.

6. Place all the vegetables in one package in the fridge container in the fridge.

7. Place the tuna in a separate zip-lock bag.

Nutrition:

Calories: 467

Total Fat: 18g

Protein: 56g

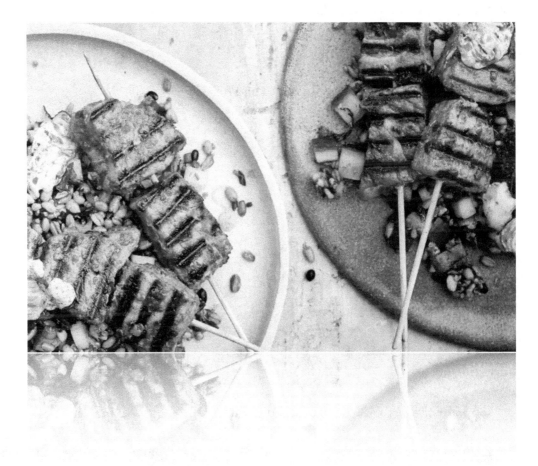

Asparagus Fries

Preparation Time: 10 minutes

Cooking Time: 10 minutes

Servings: 2

Ingredients:

- 10 medium organic asparagus spears

- 1 tbsp. of organic roasted red pepper, chopped

- ¼ cup of almond flour

- ½ tsp. of garlic powder

- ½ tsp. of smoked paprika

- 2 tbsp. of chopped parsley

- ½ cup of parmesan cheese, grated and full-fat

- 2 Organic eggs, beaten

- 3 tbsp. of mayonnaise, full-fat

Kitchen Equipment:

- oven

- food processor

- baking sheet

Directions:

1. Set the oven to 425 degrees and preheat.

2. Meanwhile, place cheese in a food processor, add garlic and parsley and pulse for 1 minute until fine mixture comes together.

3. Add almond flour, pulse for 30 seconds until just mixed, then tip the mixture into a bowl and season with paprika.

4. Break eggs into a shallow dish and whisk until beaten.

5. Working on one asparagus spear at a time, first dip into the egg mixture, then coat with the parmesan mixture and place it on a baking sheet.

6. Dip and coat more asparagus in the same manner, then arrange them on a baking sheet, 1-inch apart, and bake in the oven for 10 minutes or until asparagus is tender and nicely golden brown.

7. Meanwhile, place mayonnaise in a bowl, add red pepper and whisk until combined and chill the dip into the refrigerator until required.

8. Serve asparagus with prepared dip.

Nutrition:

Calories: 453

Fat: 33.4g

Protein: 19.1g

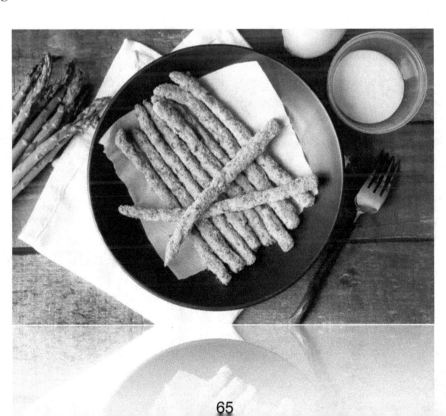

Veggie Chips

Preparation Time: 5 minutes

Cooking Time: 12 minutes

Servings: 4

Ingredients:

- 1 Large bunch of organic kale

- 1 tbsp. of seasoned salt

- 2 tbsp. of olive oil

Kitchen Equipment:

- oven

- vegetable spinner

- plastic bag

- large baking sheet

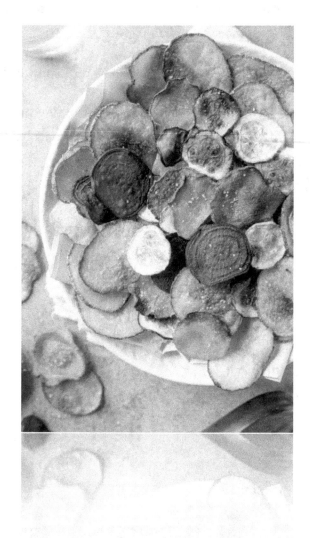

Directions:

1. Set oven to 350 degrees F.

2. Meanwhile, separate kale leaves from its stem, rinse the leaves under running water, then drain completely by using a vegetable spinner.

3. Wipe kale leaves with paper towels to remove excess water, then transfer them into a large plastic bag and add oil.

4. Seal the plastic bag, turn it upside down until kale is coated with oil and then spread kale leaves on a large baking sheet.

5. Situate the baking sheet into the oven and bake for 12 minutes or until its edges are nicely golden brown.

6. Remove baking sheet from the oven, season kale with salt and serve.

Nutrition: Calories: 163 - **Fat:** 10g - **Protein:** 2g

Coconut Shrimp

Preparation Time: 10 minutes

Cooking Time: 12 minutes

Servings: 4

Ingredients:

- 1 lb. of medium-sized shrimp (wild-caught, peeled, deveined)
- 3 tbsp. of coconut flour
- ¼ tsp. of garlic powder
- 3 Eggs (pastured, beaten)
- 1 ¾ cup of coconut flakes (unsweetened)
- 1/8 tsp. of ground black pepper
- ¼ tsp. of smoked paprika
- ¼ tsp. of sea salt

Kitchen Equipment:

- oven
- nonstick wire rack
- broiler
- parchment paper

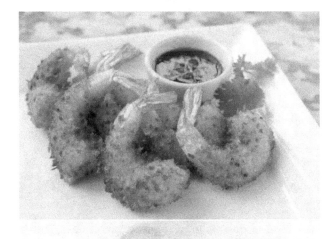

Directions:

1. Set the oven to 400 degrees F.
2. Beat eggs in a bowl and whisk until beaten, place coconut flakes in another dish, then place coconut flour in another dish, add salt, black pepper, garlic powder, and paprika and stir until mixed.
3. Working on one piece at a time, dredge a shrimp into the coconut flour mix, then dip into egg, and dredge with coconut flake until evenly coated.
4. Take a non-stick wire rack, line it with a baking sheet, then spray with oil and place coated shrimps on it in a single layer.
5. Place the wire rack containing shrimps into the oven, bake for 4 minutes, then flip the shrimps and continue baking for 5 to 6 minutes or until thoroughly cooked and firm.
6. Then switch on the broiler and bake the shrimps for 2 minutes or until lightly golden.
7. When done, let shrimps cooled, place them on a baking sheet in a single layer, then cover the shrimps with parchment sheet, layer with remaining shrimps and freeze until hard.
8. Then transfer shrimps into a freezer bag and store in the freezer for up to 3 months.
9. When ready to serve, reheat the shrimps at 350 degrees F for 2 to 3 minutes until hot.

Nutrition: Calories: 443 - **Fat:** 30g - **Protein:** 31g

Sausage Stuffed Zucchini Boats

Preparation Time: 10 minutes

Cooking Time: 30 minutes

Servings: 4

Ingredients:

- 4 Medium zucchinis

- 1 lb. of ground Italian pork sausage, pastured

- 1 ½ tsp. of sea salt

- 1/3 cup of medium white onion, peeled, diced

- 1 tbsp. of minced garlic

- 1 tsp. of Italian seasoning

- 14.5 oz. of diced tomatoes

- 1/3 cup of grated parmesan cheese, full-fat

- 2 tbsp. of avocado oil, divided

- 1 cup of mozzarella cheese, full-fat, shredded

Kitchen Equipment:

- oven

- baking sheet

- parchment paper

- skillet pan

- aluminum foil

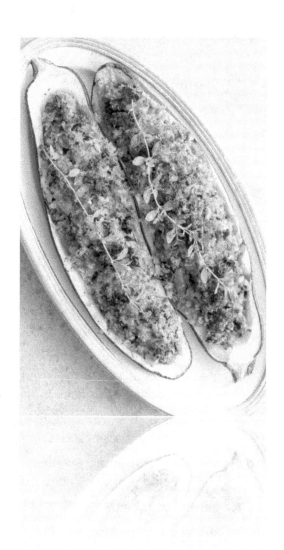

Directions:

1. Set the oven to 400 degrees F and let preheat. Meanwhile, cut each zucchini in half, lengthwise, then make well in the center by scooping out the centers by using a spoon.

2. Take a baking sheet, line it with parchment sheet, place zucchini halves on it, cut side up, drizzle with 1 tablespoon oil and season with salt.

3. Situate the baking sheet into the oven and bake for 15 to 20 minutes or until soft. Meanwhile, take a large skillet pan, place it over medium-high heat, add remaining oil and when hot, add onions and cook for 10 minutes until nicely brown.

4. Add sausage, stir well and cook for 5 minutes or until brown.

5. Then move sausage to one side of the pan, add garlic to the other side, cook for 1 minute or until fragrant and then mix into the sausage.

6. Remove pan from the heat, season sausage with Italian seasoning, add tomatoes and parmesan cheese, stir well and taste to adjust seasoning.

7. When zucchini halves are roasted, pat dry with paper towels, then stuff with sausage mixture.

8. Top stuffed zucchini with mozzarella cheese and bake for 5 to 10 minutes or until cheese melts and the top is nicely golden brown.

9. Let zucchini boats cool down, then wrap each zucchini boat with an aluminum foil and freeze in the freezer.

10. When ready to serve, thaw the zucchini boat and reheat at 350 degrees F for 3 to 4 minutes until hot.

Nutrition:

Calories: 582

Fat: 44g

Protein: 29g

Garlicky Green Beans

Gluten Free, Nut Free, Vegetarian

Preparation Time: 10 minutes

Cooking Time: 10 minutes

Servings: 4

Ingredients:

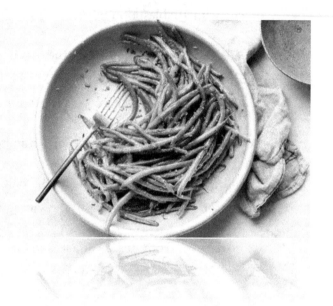

- 1-pound of green beans, stemmed
- 2 tablespoons of olive oil
- 1 teaspoon of minced garlic
- Sea salt
- Freshly ground black pepper
- ¼ cup of freshly grated Parmesan cheese

Kitchen Equipment:

- oven
- baking sheet
- aluminum foil
- large bowl

Directions:

1. Preheat the oven to 425°F.
2. Put aluminum foil in a baking sheet and set aside.
3. In a large bowl, toss together the green beans, olive oil, and garlic.
4. Season the beans lightly.
5. Arrange the beans on the baking sheet and roast them until they are tender and lightly browned, stirring them once, about 10 minutes.
6. Serve topped with the Parmesan cheese.

Nutrition: Calories: 104 - **Fat:** 9g - **Protein:** 4g

Bacon-Artichoke Omelet

Gluten Free, Nut Free

Preparation Time: 10 minutes

Cooking Time: 10 minutes

Servings: 4

Ingredients:

- 6 eggs, beaten

- 2 tablespoons of heavy (whipping) cream

- 8 bacon slices (cooked and chopped)

- 1 tablespoon of olive oil

- ¼ cup of chopped onion

- ½ cup of chopped artichoke hearts (canned, packed in water)

- Sea salt

- Freshly ground black pepper

Kitchen Equipment:

- small bowl

- large skillet

Directions:

1. Beat together the eggs, heavy cream, and bacon until well blended, and set aside. Situate a large skillet over medium-high heat and pour the olive oil.

2. Sauté the onion until tender, about 3 minutes. Pour the egg mixture into the skillet, swirling it for 1 minute.

3. Cook the omelet, tilt pan to let the uncooked egg flow underneath, for 2 minutes.

4. Sprinkle the artichoke hearts on top and flip the omelet.

5. Cook for 4 minutes more, until the egg is firm.

6. Flip the omelet over again so the artichoke hearts are on top.

7. Remove from the heat, cut the omelet into quarters, and season with salt and black pepper.

8. Transfer the omelet to plates and serve.

Nutrition:

Calories: 435

Fat: 39g

Protein: 17

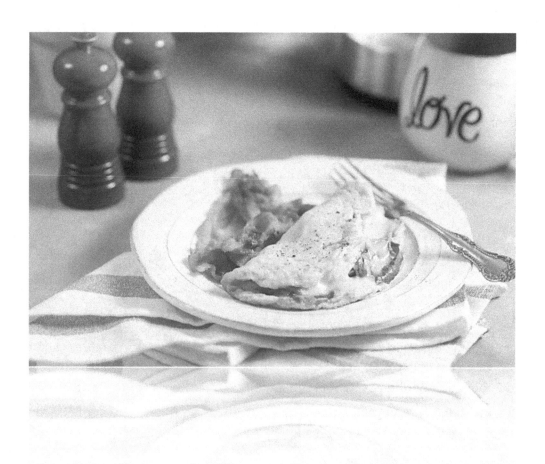

Rainbow Mason Jar Salad

Preparation Time: 10 minutes

Cooking Time: 30 minutes

Servings: 1

Ingredients:

For the Salad:

- ½ cup of Arugula (fresh)

- 2 Medium radishes (sliced)

- ¼ Medium yellow squash (spiralized)

- ¼ cup of Butternut squash (peeled, cubed)

- ¼ cup of Fresh blueberries

- 1 tbsp. of Avocado oil

The Dressing:

- ¼ Medium avocado (peeled, cubed)

- 2 tbsp. of Avocado oil

- 1 tbsp. of Apple cider vinegar

- 1 tbsp. of Filtered water

- 1 tbsp. of Cilantro leaves

- ¼ tsp. of Salt

Kitchen Equipment:

- oven

- baking sheet

- blender

Directions:

1. Set the oven to 350 degrees F.

2. Then place cubes of butternut squash in a bowl, drizzle with oil, toss until well coated and then spread evenly on a baking sheet.

3. Situate the baking sheet into the oven and bake for 30 minutes or until tender.

4. Meanwhile, prepare the salad dressing and for this, place all the ingredients for the dressing in a blender and pulse for 1 to 2 minutes or until smooth, set aside until required.

5. When the butternut squash is baked, take out the baking sheet from the oven and let squash cool for 15 minutes.

6. Then take a 32-ounce mason jar, pour in the prepared dressing, layer with radish, and top with roasted butternut squash, squash noodles, berries, and arugula.

7. Seal the jar and store in the refrigerator for up to 5 days.

Nutrition:

Calories: 516

Fat: 49g

Protein: 2g

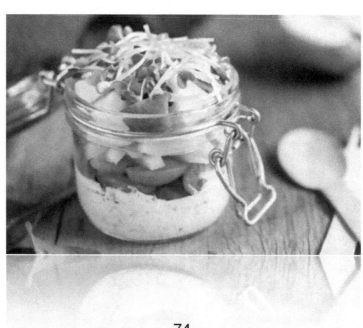

Creamy Chicken Pot Pie Soup

Preparation Time: 20 minutes

Cooking Time: 35 minutes

Servings: 6

Ingredients:

- 2 tablespoons of extra-virgin olive oil (divided)

- 1 pound (454 g) of skinless chicken breast (cut into ½-inch chunks)

- 1 cup of mushrooms (quartered)

- 2 celery stalks (chopped)

- 1 onion (chopped)

- 1 tablespoon of garlic (minced)

- 5 cups of low-sodium chicken broth

- 1 cup of green beans (chopped)

- ¼ cup of cream cheese

- 1 cup of heavy whipping cream

- 1 tablespoon of fresh thyme (chopped)

- Salt and black pepper (to taste)

Kitchen Equipment:

- stockpot

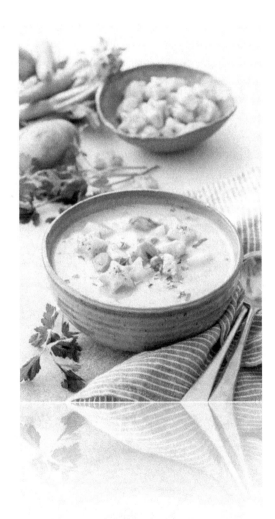

Directions:

1. Cook the olive oil in a stockpot over medium-high heat until shimmering.

2. Add the chicken chunks to the pot and sauté for 10 minutes or until well browned.

3. Transfer the chicken to a plate. Set aside until ready to use.

4. Cook the remaining olive oil in the stockpot over medium-high heat.

5. Add the mushrooms, celery, onion, and garlic to the pot and sauté for 6 minutes or until fork-tender.

6. Pour the chicken broth over, then add the cooked chicken chunks to the pot.

7. Stir to mix well, and bring the soup to a boil.

8. Set heat to low, and simmer for 15 minutes or until the vegetables are soft and the internal temperature of the chicken reaches at least 165°F (74°C).

9. Mix in the green beans, cream cheese, cream, thyme, salt, and black pepper, then simmer for 3 minutes more.

10. Remove the soup from the stockpot and serve hot.

Nutrition:

Calories: 338

Total fat: 26.1g

Fiber: 2.2g

Chicken Egg Soup

Preparation Time: 10 minutes

Cooking Time: 20 minutes

Servings: 6

Ingredients:

- 4 large eggs

- 2 quarts of chicken or vegetable stock

- 1 tbsp. of grated turmeric

- 1 tbsp. of grated ginger

- 6 tbsp. of extra-virgin olive oil

- 2 tbsp. of coconut aminos

- 2 tbsp. of freshly chopped cilantro

- 1 tsp. of salt or to taste

- 2 cloves of garlic (minced)

- 2 cups of sliced brown mushrooms

- 4 cups of chopped Swiss chard/spinach

- 1 small chili pepper (sliced)

- 2 medium spring onions (sliced)

- freshly ground black pepper to taste

Kitchen Equipment:

- stock

- bowl

Directions:

1. Transfer the chicken stock in a large pot. Apply medium heat until it starts to simmer.

2. Put the turmeric, ginger, chili pepper, mushroom, coconut aminos, and char stalks into the pot.

3. Allow it to simmer for 5 more minutes.

4. Include the sliced chard leaves and allow it to cook for another minute in a separate bowl, whisk the eggs and then pour them carefully into the soup.

5. Stir constantly until the egg is cooked.

6. Add the chopped cilantro and spring onions to the pot.

7. Add salt and pepper to taste.

8. Serve with a drizzle of extra virgin olive oil. You can store this for five days in an airtight container in the fridge.

Nutrition:

Calories: 255

Protein: 10.8g

Net carbohydrates: 2.9g

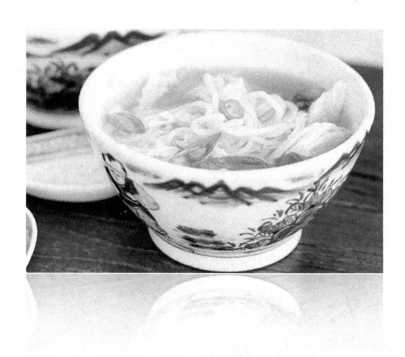

Coconut Bars

Preparation Time: 10 minutes

Cooking Time: 0 minute

Servings: 20

Ingredients:

- 3 cups of unsweetened shredded coconut

- 1 cup of coconut oil

- ¼ cup of liquid sweetener of choice

Kitchen Equipment:

- pan

- parchment paper

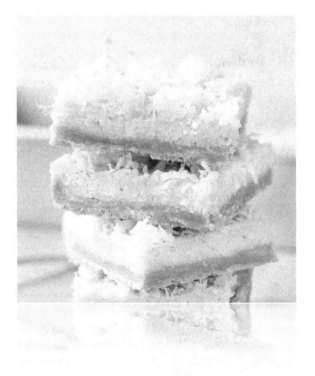

Directions:

1. Line a pan with a layer of parchment paper.

2. Combine the ingredients to make a thick batter.

3. Pour into the pan and freeze until firm.

4. Cut into squares and store until you want a delicious snack.

Nutrition:

Protein Counts: 2g

Total Fats: 11g

Calories: 108

Coconut Cranberry Crack Bars

Preparation Time: 15 minutes

Cooking Time: 0 minute

Servings: 20

Ingredients:

- 2 ½ cups of unsweetened shredded coconut flakes

- ½ cup of unsweetened cranberries

- ¼ cup of monk fruit sweetened maple syrup/agave/pure maple syrup

- 1 cup of melted coconut oil

Kitchen Equipment:

- 8x8/8x10 baking tray

- blender or food processor

- pan

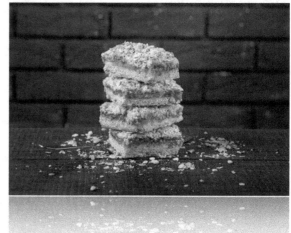

Directions:

1. Use a high-speed blender/food processor to combine the berries and coconut, pulsing until it's crumbly.

2. Combine all of the fixings until thoroughly mixed.

3. Transfer the batter into the pan and refrigerate until firm.

4. Slice into bars and add a bar of optional chocolate to your liking. They're okay in the fridge for up to two months.

Nutrition:

Protein Counts: 2g - **Total Fats:** 9g - **Calories:** 98

Low-Carb Cheesecake

Preparation Time: 10 minutes

Cooking Time: 20 minutes

Servings: 5

Ingredients:

- 8 oz. of room temp full-fat cream cheese

- 2 Large eggs

- 1 ½ tsp. of granulated stevia/erythritol blend

- ¼ tsp. of pure vanilla extract

- ¼ tsp. of pure almond extract

Kitchen Equipment:

- oven

- muffin tin cups

- cupcake liners

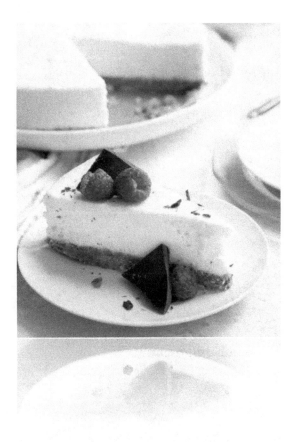

Directions:

1. Warm the oven to 325° Fahrenheit.

2. Prepare five muffin tin cups using cupcake liners.

3. Beat the cream cheese until it's creamy smooth, whisk in the eggs, and the rest of the fixings.

4. Dump the batter into the muffin tins.

5. Set the timer (15–20 minutes) and bake until the cheesecakes are puffy but still wobbly in the center.

6. Cool to room temperature before placing it in the refrigerator to chill for two hours before serving.

Nutrition: Protein: 4g **Total Fats:** 17g - **Calories** 181

Coconut Bars

Preparation Time: 10 minutes

Cooking Time: 15 minutes

Servings: 12

Ingredients:

- 1 tsp. of vanilla extract

- ½ cup of almond meal

- ¾ cup of granulated no calorie sucralose sweetener

- ¼ cup of melted butter

- 2 eggs

- 2 8 oz. pack of softened cream cheese

Kitchen Equipment:

- oven

- muffin cups

- paper liners

Directions:

1. Prepare your oven to 350 degrees F. Also, prepare 12 muffin cups by lining them with paper liners.

2. Grab a bowl and put your butter and almond meal in it.

3. Using a spoon, take the almond meal mixture and put into the bottom of the muffin cup.

4. Press them down with the flat of the spoon to form a crust.

5. In a separate bowl, add vanilla extract, cream cheese, sucralose sweetener, and eggs.

6. Set an electric mixer to medium and combine the vanilla extract mixture until you get a smooth consistency.

7. Using a spoon, add this mixture to the top of the muffin cups.

8. Pop the muffin cups in the oven and bake until the center of the mixture is slightly set for no more than 17 minutes.

9. Now, you have your cupcakes. Set them aside to cool.

10. When they are safe enough to hold again, put them in your refrigerator. They should stay there 8 hours until the next day, when you can serve them.

Nutrition: **Calories:** 209 - **Protein:** 4.9g - **Fat:** 20g

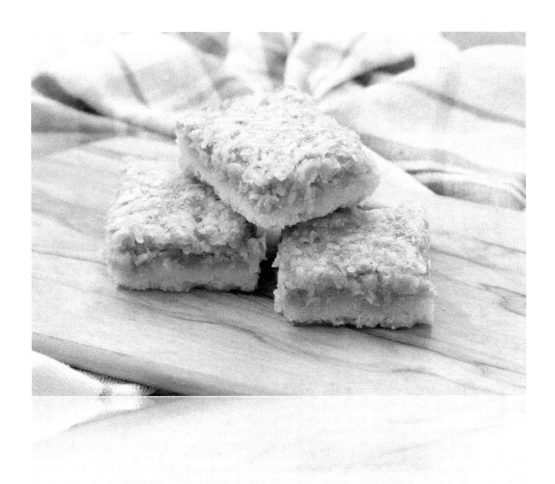

Cocoa Mug Cake

Preparation Time: 5 minutes

Cooking Time: 1 minute

Servings: 2

Ingredients:

- 2 tbsp. of melted coconut oil

- 6 tbsp. of almond flour

- 2 eggs

- 2 tbsp. of cocoa powder (unsweetened)

- Pinch salt

- 2 tsp. of natural sweetener (low-calorie)

- ½ tsp. of baking powder

Kitchen Equipment:

- small bowl

- electric mixer

- 2 mugs

- microwave

Directions:

1. Get a small bowl and add salt, almond flour, baking powder, cocoa powder, natural sweetener.

2. Into a second bowl, crack the eggs and beat with an electric mixer until you have a fluffy liquid.

3. Next, add coconut oil and stir properly.

4. Pour this egg mixture into the previous bowl containing baking powder.

5. Using a fork, whisk this mixture.

6. Prepare 2 mugs that are safe to go in a microwave by oiling them lightly.

7. Pour the mixture in your bowl into these cups. Let there be some space at the top of the cups: at least, 1 inch. This is so that the cake will have room to rise without spilling over.

8. Adjust the microwave to high and place the cups inside it for 1 minute.

9. Take the cups out and check if the cakes have set and are done enough to serve. If not, put them back in the microwave.

10. Check the cakes every 10 seconds until you're satisfied that they are ready. That is, the center of the cakes should not be runny.

Nutrition: Calories: 338 - **Protein:** 12.3g - **Fat:** 30.9g

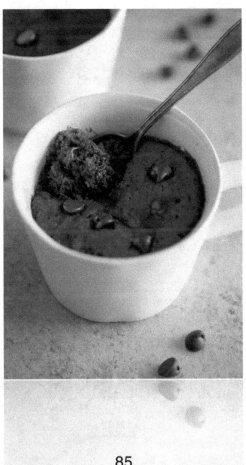

Dark Chocolate Espresso Paleo and Keto Mug Cake

Preparation Time: 5 minutes

Cooking Time: 2 minutes

Servings: 1

Ingredients:

- 1 tbsp. of brewed espresso

- 4 oz. of dark chocolate chips

- 1 egg

- 1 tbsp. of coconut oil

- Pinch baking soda

- 2 tbsp. of water

- 1 tbsp. of coconut flour

- 1 tbsp. of almond flour (blanched)

Kitchen Equipment:

- mug

- microwave

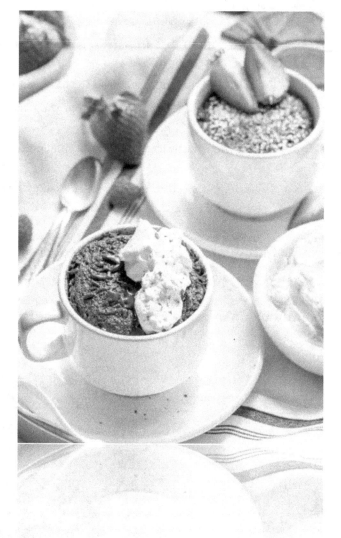

Directions:

1. Get a mug that can safely go into a microwave and put both the coconut oil and chocolate chips in it.

2. Next, add baking soda, water, coconut flour, and almond flour to the coconut oil mixture in the mug.

3. You may now place the mug in the microwave and cook for about 1 minute and 30 seconds. The cake should be cooked through at this point.

4. Let the mug sit for 2 minutes before you dig in.

Nutrition: Calories: 793 - **Protein:** 14g - **Fat:** 52.2g

Lemon Poppy Seed Muffins

Preparation Time: 15 minutes

Cooking Time: 15 minutes

Servings: 8

Ingredients:

- 2 tbsp. of heavy whipping cream

- 1/3 cup of natural sweetener, low-calorie

- ½ tsp. of vanilla extract

- ¼ cup of almond flour

- 2 tbsp. of sour cream

- ¼ cup of coconut flour

- 3 tbsp. of butter

- 1 tbsp. of poppy seeds

- 3 eggs

- 1 lemon zest

- ¼ tsp. of xanthan gum

- ½ tsp. of baking powder

- ½ tsp. of salt

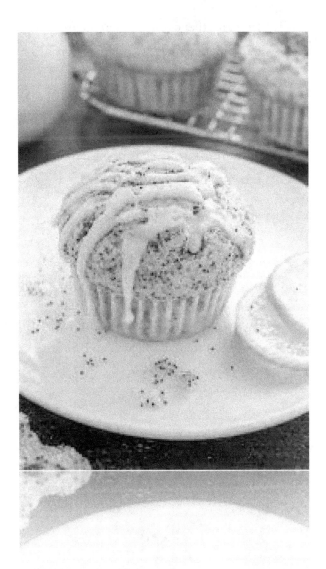

Kitchen Equipment:

- oven

- muffin tin

- parchment paper

- muffin liners

- small bowl

- electric mixer

Directions:

1. Prepare the oven to 350 degrees F. Prepare a muffin tin by oiling and lining it with parchment paper. Make the paper into muffin liners.

2. In a small bowl, add your poppy seeds, natural sweetener, xanthan gum, coconut flour, lemon zest, almond flour, baking powder, and salt. Mix well.

3. Now, break your eggs open into a different bowl and beat with an electric mixer. Adjust the mixer to high speed and beat the eggs for 2 straight minutes.

4. Next, you should add vanilla extract, butter, the mixture in the previous small bowl, and butter.

5. Stir this mixture slowly but properly, until you get a thick yet smooth batter.

6. Turn this into your muffin tin and let it bake in your oven for 20 minutes. The top of the muffins should be brown and an inserted toothpick should come out clean.

7. Let cool and serve!

Nutrition:

Calories: 116

Protein: 3.6g

Fat: 10.7g

Chapter 5. Recipes from France

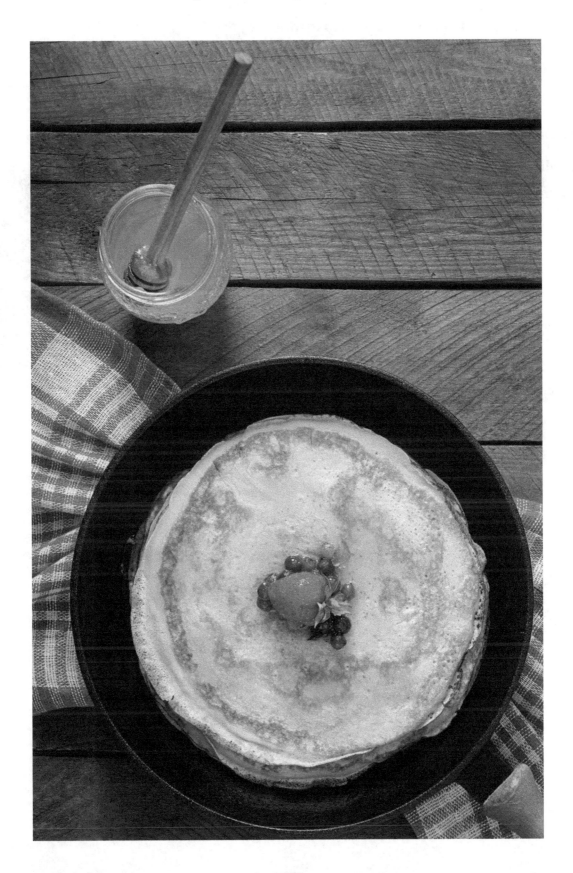

Stuffed Basil- Asiago Mushrooms

Preparation Time: 10 minutes

Cooking Time: 35 minutes

Servings: 4

Ingredients:

- 24 Portobello mushrooms (remove the stems)

- ½ cup of mayonnaise

- ¾ cup of Asiago cheese(shredded)

- 1/3 cup of basil leaves (remove the stems)

- ¼ tsp. of white pepper

- 12 cherry tomatoes (halved)

Kitchen Equipment:

- oven

- baking dish

- food processor

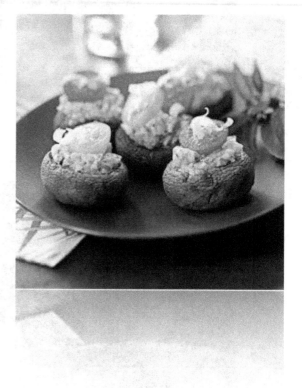

Directions:

1. Preheat your oven at 150 degrees Celsius. Grease a baking dish with cooking spray.

2. Arrange the mushroom caps in the dish.

3. Bake the mushrooms for ten minutes.

4. Combine Asiago cheese, mayonnaise, pepper, and basil in a food processor. Mix well.

5. Pour the mushroom caps with the cheese and basil mixture.

6. Top each mushroom cap with half a tomato.

7. Bake for ten minutes.

8. Serve warm.

Nutrition: Calories: 36.6 - **Protein:** 2.3g - **Fat:** 3.3g

Cheese and Zucchini Roulades

Preparation Time: 10 minutes

Cooking Time: 25 minutes

Servings: 6

Ingredients:

- 1 cup of ricotta cheese

- ¼ cup of parmesan cheese (grated)

- 2 tbsps. of basil (minced)

- 1 tbsp. of capers

- 1 ½ tbsp. of Greek olives (chopped)

- 1 tsp. of lemon zest (grated)

- 2 tbsps. of lemon juice

- 1/8 tsp. of pepper

- 1/4 tsp. of salt

- 4 zucchinis

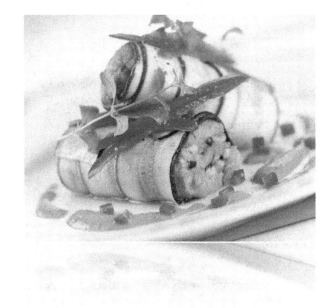

Kitchen Equipment:

- grill rack

Directions:

1. Combine the first nine listed ingredients in a bowl.

2. Slice the zucchinis into twenty-four slices lengthwise.

3. Grease a grill rack with cooking spray.

4. Cook the slices of zucchini for three minutes.

5. Add one tbsp. of the ricotta cheese mixture on one end of the zucchini slices.

6. Roll up the slices. Secure using toothpicks.

7. Serve immediately.

Nutrition: Calories: 29.4 - **Protein:** 3.5g - **Fat:** 1.6g

Corned Beef and Cauliflower Hash

Preparation Time: 5 minutes

Cooking Time: 15 minutes

Servings: 4

Ingredients:

- 2 cups of chopped raw cauliflower

- ½ cup of onion (chopped)

- 2 cups of chopped corned beef

- 1 tablespoon of extra-virgin olive oil

- Pepper and salt to taste

Kitchen Equipment:

- medium-sized sauté pan

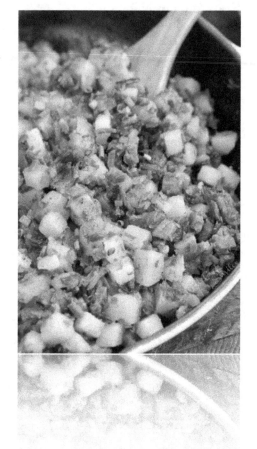

Directions:

1. Over moderate heat in a medium-sized sauté pan; heat the olive oil until hot.

2. Carefully, add the corned beef and cook until the fat renders out, for a couple of minutes.

3. Add the raw cauliflower and continue to cook until caramelized, for 6 to 8 minutes, stirring every now and then.

4. Add and cook the onions until slightly browned and softened, for more 5 minutes.

5. Season with pepper and salt to taste.

6. Serve immediately and enjoy.

Nutrition:

Calories: 275 - **Total Fat:** 19g - **Total Carbohydrates:** 4.4g

Artichoke and Spinach Stuffed Mushrooms

Preparation Time: 10 minutes

Cooking Time: 40 minutes

Servings: 6

Ingredients:

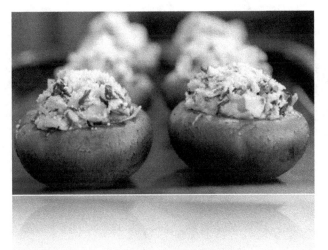

- 3 ounces of cream cheese
- ½ cup of mayonnaise
- 1 cup of sour cream
- ¾ tsp. of garlic salt
- 1 can of artichoke hearts (chopped)
- 10 ounces of spinach (chopped)
- 1/3 cup of mozzarella cheese (shredded)
- 3 tbsps. of parmesan cheese (shredded)
- 30 large mushrooms (remove the stems)

Kitchen Equipment:

- oven
- aluminum foil
- baking tray

Directions:

1. Preheat your oven at 200 degrees Celsius.
2. Combine the first four listed ingredients in a bowl.
3. Add spinach, artichoke, three tbsps. of parmesan cheese, and mozzarella cheese.
4. Arrange the mushrooms on a large aluminum foil-lined baking tray.
5. Add one tbsp. of the filling into the mushroom caps.
6. Sprinkle remaining parmesan cheese from the top. Bake for twenty minutes.

Nutrition: Calories: 52.2 - **Protein:** 2.6g - **Fat:** 5.6g

Pork Belly Cracklings

Preparation Time: 10 minutes

Cooking Time: 80 minutes

Servings: 6

Ingredients:

- 3 pounds of pork belly (with skin)

- 2 cups of water

- 4 tbsp of Cajun seasoning

Kitchen Equipment:

- cast-iron pot

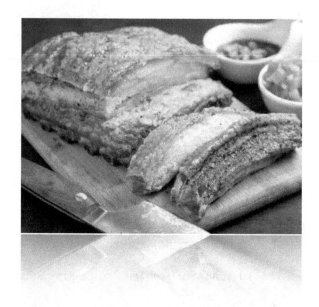

Directions:

1. Keep the pork belly in the refrigerator for 40 minutes.

2. Cut the pork into cubes of three-fourth inch.

3. Fill a cast-iron pot with one-fourth portion of water.

4. Add one tsp. of Cajun seasoning.

5. Boil the water.

6. Add the cubes of pork belly.

7. Cook for twenty minutes.

8. Cover the pot once fat begins to pop and sizzle.

9. Cook for fifteen minutes.

10. Drain the pork cracklings.

11. Sprinkle remaining seasoning from the top.

12. Serve immediately.

Nutrition: Calories: 210.3 - **Protein:** 16.5g - **Fat:** 16.6g

Lemon Fat Bombs

Preparation Time: 10 minutes

Cooking Time: 50 minutes

Servings: 4

Ingredients:

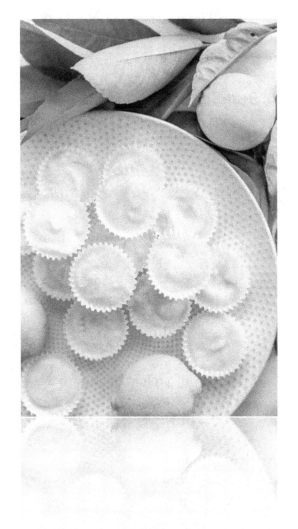

- 1 cup of shredded coconut (dry)

- ¼ cup of coconut oil

- 3 tbsp. of erythritol sweetener (powdered)

- 1 tbsp. of lemon zest

- 1 pinch of salt

Kitchen Equipment:

- blender

Directions:

1. Add the coconut in a high-power blender.

2. Blend until creamy for fifteen minutes.

3. Add sweetener, coconut oil, salt, and lemon zest.

4. Blend for two minutes.

5. Fill small muffin cups with the coconut mixture.

6. Chill in the refrigerator for 30 minutes.

Nutrition:

Calories: 69.9 - **Protein:** 0.5g - **Fat:** 7.9g

Crustless Quiche Lorraine

Preparation Time: 5 minutes

Cooking Time: 40 minutes

Servings: 4

Ingredients:

- 8 Slices of bacon, chopped

- 4 Eggs

- ¼ tsp. of salt

- ¼ tsp. of nutmeg

- 1 ½ cup of heavy whipping cream

- 1 1/3 cup of Swiss cheese, shredded

- ¼ tsp. of ground black pepper

- 1 cup of water

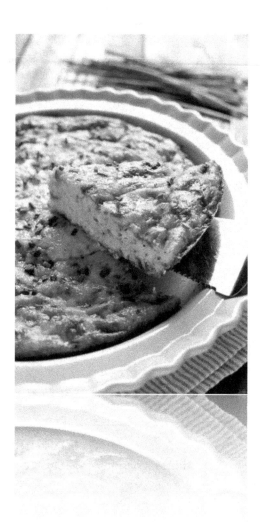

Kitchen Equipment:

- instant pot

- 6-inch baking dish

- broiler

Directions:

1. Turn on the instant pot, click the 'sauté/simmer' button, wait until hot and stir in the bacon.

2. Cook chopped bacon for 5 minutes or more until crispy, then transfer it to a plate lined with paper towels and set aside.

3. Break eggs in a bowl, add cream, season with salt, black pepper, and nutmeg and whisk until combined.

4. Take a 6-inch baking dish, place 1 cup of cheese in the bottom, then top with bacon and evenly pour in the egg mixture.

5. Press the 'keep warm' button, pour water in the instant pot, insert a trivet stand and place baking dish on it.

6. Seal the instant pot, then click the 'manual' button, press '+/-' to select cooking time to 25 minutes and adjust at high-pressure setting; when the pressure kicks in the pot, it will start.

7. When the timer rings, select the 'keep warm' button, release pressure naturally for 10 minutes, then lightly open the lid to release pressure.

8. Meanwhile, switch on the broiler and let it preheat.

9. Take out the baking dish, spread the remaining cheese on top, then place it under the broiler and broil for 5 minutes or until the cheese melts and the top is nicely browned.

10. When done, turn the dish over a plate to take out the quiche, then cut into slices and serve.

Nutrition:

Calories: 572

Fat: 52.54g

Protein: 22g

Cheesy Ham Quiche

Preparation Time: 10 minutes

Cooking Time: 40 minutes

Servings: 6

Ingredients:

- 8 Eggs

- 1 cup of Zucchini

- ½ cup of heavy Cream

- 1 cup of ham

- 1 tsp. of mustard

- A dash of Salt

Kitchen Equipment:

- stove

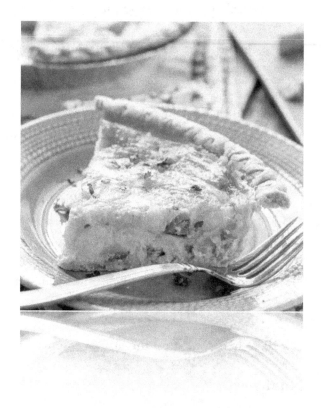

Directions:

1. Prepare your stove to 375 degrees and get out a pie plate for your quiche.

2. Prepare the zucchini by shredding it into small pieces.

3. Then take a paper towel and gently squeeze out the excess moisture. This will help to avoid a soggy quiche.

4. Put the zucchini into your pie plate along with the cooked ham pieces and your cheese.

5. Whisk the seasonings, cream, and eggs together before pouring it over the top.

6. Place the dish into your stove for about forty minutes. By the end of this time, the egg should be cooked through, and you will be able to insert a knife into the center and have it come out clean.

7. If the quiche is cooked to your liking, take the dish from the oven and allow it to chill slightly before slicing and serving.

Nutrition: Fats: 25g - **Carbs:** 2g - **Protein** 20g

Loaded Cauliflower Rice

Preparation Time: 10 minutes

Cooking Time: 30 minutes

Servings: 4

Ingredients:

- 1 head of cauliflower

- 1 cup of cheddar cheese

- 1 lb. of bacon

- ½ cup of chives

- A dash of salt

Kitchen Equipment:

- grilling pan

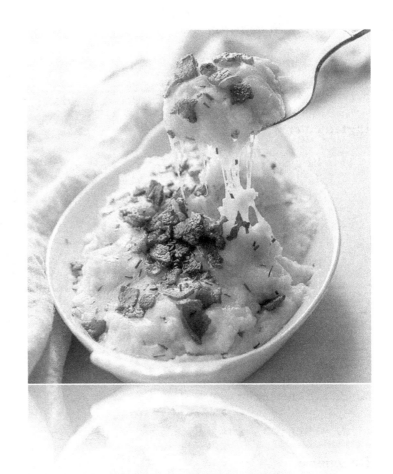

Directions:

1. Rice your cauliflower.

2. Heat the grilling pan over a moderate temperature and cook the bacon for four or five minutes on either side.

3. Place your cauliflower rice into a microwave-safe bowl and sprinkle your shredded cheese over the top. When this is set, go ahead and pop the bowl into the microwave for a minute and allow for the rice to cook through and the cheese to melt.

4. Topped the dish off with your bacon pieces and season to your liking.

Nutrition:

Fats: 10g - **Carbs:** 5g - **Proteins:** 5g

Cheesy Chive Omelet

Preparation Time: 10 minutes

Cooking Time: 30 minutes

Servings: 2

Ingredients:

- 4 Eggs

- 1 cup of cheddar cheese

- A dash of salt

- 1 tbsp. of butter

- 1 tbsp. of chives

- ¼ cup of water

- A dash of pepper

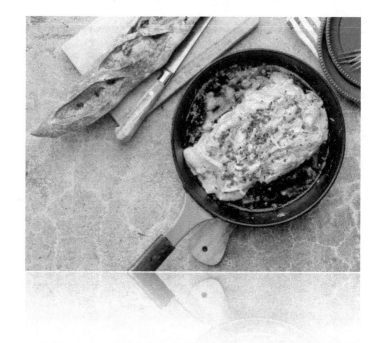

Kitchen Equipment:

- frying pan

Directions:

1. Put frying pan over a moderate temperature. It is important to make sure the surface is hot before doing anything.

2. When the pan is heating up, combine the water, eggs, and seasoning.

3. Carefully pour the mixture into your hot pan and wait several minutes.

4. Lift your pan a bit to create an even omelet.

5. After several minutes, sprinkle some of the cheese over half of your omelet.

6. Use thin spatula to turn half of the omelet over.

7. Sprinkle the rest of the cheese over the top of the omelet and continue to cook until it is browned or cooked to your liking.

8. Drizzle some pepper and salt over the top for some additional flavor.

Nutrition: Fats: - 15g - **Carbs:** 2g - **Protein** 8g

Buttery Garlic Steak

Preparation Time: 10 minutes

Cooking Time: 30 minutes

Servings: 4

Ingredients:

- 1 lb. of steak

- 5 tbsp. of grass-fed butter

- 5 tbsp. of garlic cloves

- ¼ cup of parsley

- A dash salt

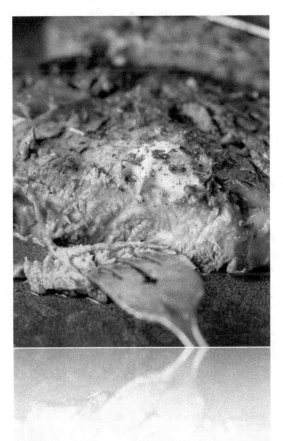

Kitchen Equipment:

- heavy duty skillet

Directions:

1. Pat the steak down then seasoned it with pepper and salt on both sides. Be generous with your seasoning!

2. Cook the steak in a heavy-duty skillet over a moderate temperature and sear both sides for about 3 minutes. If you like your steak cooked past medium-rare, leave it on longer.

3. When the steak is cooked to your liking, remove it from the pan and set to the side.

To make garlic butter:

1. Lower the heat in your skillet and begin melting your butter.

2. Once the butter has been liquefied, you will next add in the garlic and cook for an additional minute.

3. When the garlic turns a golden color, take the pan away from the heat.

4. Drizzle your butter sauce over the top until the steak becomes completely coated.

5. As a final touch, garnish with some fresh parsley and enjoy your dinner.

Nutrition:Fats: 25g **Carbs:** 2g - **Protein** 25g

Beef Stew

Preparation Time: 5 minutes

Cooking Time: 80 minutes

Servings: 4

Ingredients:

- 3 ½ lbs. of beef, grass-fed (diced)

- 3 stalks of celery (chopped)

- 1 leek (white part only)

- 15 oz. of diced tomatoes

- ¾ cup of spinach leaves (fresh)

- 3 carrots (chopped into large rounds)

- 1 tbsp. of chopped ginger

- ½ tbsp. of minced garlic

- 1 ½ tsp. of salt

- ¾ tsp. of ground black pepper

- 2 tsp. of dried rosemary

- 2 tsp. of dried thyme

- 2 tsp. of dried oregano

- 2 tbsp. of apple cider vinegar

- 2 tbsp. of avocado oil

- 1 ½ cup of beef broth (grass-fed)

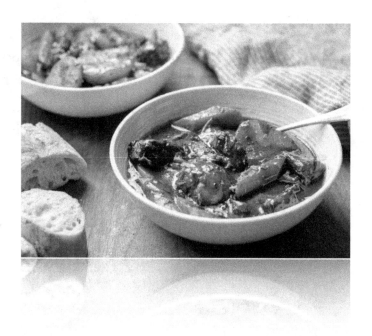

Kitchen Equipment:

- frying pan

- slow cooker

- plastic wrap

- microwave

Directions:

1. Take a frying pan, place it over medium heat, add oil and when hot, add beef and cook for 3 to 5 minutes or until light brown.

2. Transfer beef into a slow cooker, add remaining ingredients, except for spinach and stir until mixed.

3. Switch on the slow cooker, shut it with lid and cook for 5 to 8 hours at low heat setting until thoroughly cooked.

4. When beef cooking is about to finish, place spinach in a heatproof bowl, cover with plastic wrap and microwave for 2 minutes until steamed.

5. When beef is cooked, taste to adjust seasoning, add spinach, and stir until just mixed and let cool.

6. Divide beef evenly between four glass containers, then seal the lid and keep in cooling for up to 5 days or freeze for up to 2 months.

7. When ready to serve, thaw the stew at room temperature and then reheat the beef stew in its glass container in the microwave for 2 to 3 minutes or until hot.

8. Serve the stew with cauliflower rice.

Nutrition:

Calories: 553 - **Fat:** 36.9g - **Protein:** 17.5g

Golden Rosti

Gluten Free, Nut Free

Preparation Time: 15 minutes

Cooking Time: 15 minutes

Servings: 8

Ingredients:

- 8 bacon slices (chopped)
- 1 cup of shredded acorn squash
- 1 cup of shredded raw celeriac
- 2 tablespoons of grated or shredded Parmesan cheese
- 2 teaspoons of minced garlic
- 1 teaspoon of chopped fresh thyme
- Sea salt
- Freshly ground black pepper
- 2 tablespoons of butter

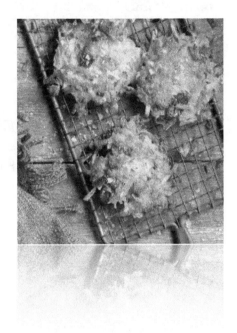

Kitchen Equipment:

- large skillet

Directions:

1. Cook the bacon in a large skillet over medium-high heat for about 5 minutes.
2. While the bacon is cooking, in a large bowl, mix together the squash, celeriac, Parmesan cheese, garlic, and thyme.
3. Season the mixture generously and set aside.
4. Remove the cooked bacon with a slotted spoon to the rosti mixture and stir to incorporate.
5. Remove all but 2 tablespoons of bacon fat from the skillet and add the butter.
6. Adjust the heat to medium-low and transfer the rosti mixture to the skillet and spread it out evenly to form a large round patty about 1 inch thick.
7. Cook until the bottom of the rosti is golden brown and crisp, about 5 minutes.
8. Flip the rosti over and cook until the other side is crispy and the middle is cooked through, about 5 minutes more.
9. Remove the skillet from the heat and cut the rosti into 8 pieces.
10. Serve.

Nutrition: Calories: 171 - **Fat:** 15g - **Protein:** 5g

Beef and Pumpkin Stew

Preparation Time: 15 minutes

Cooking Time: 75 minutes

Servings: 6

Ingredients:

- 3 tablespoons of extra-virgin olive oil (divided)

- 1 (2-pound / 907-g) beef chuck roast (cut into 1-inch chunks)

- ½ teaspoon of salt

- ¼ teaspoon of freshly ground black pepper

- ¼ cup of apple cider vinegar

- ½ sweet onion (chopped)

- 1 cup of diced tomatoes

- 1 teaspoon of dried thyme

- 1½ cups pumpkin (cut into 1-inch chunks)

- 2 cups of beef broth

- 2 teaspoons of minced garlic

- 1 tablespoon of chopped fresh parsley (for garnish)

Kitchen Equipment:

- slow cooker

- nonstick skillet

Directions:

1. Grease the insert of the slow cooker with olive oil.

2. Heat the remaining olive oil in a nonstick skillet.

3. Add the beef to the skillet, and sprinkle salt and pepper to season.

4. Cook the beef for 7 minutes or until well browned.

5. Flip the beef halfway through the cooking time.

6. Put the cooked beef into the slow cooker, then add the remaining ingredients, except for the parsley, to the slow cooker.

7. Stir to mix well.

8. Seal close the slow cooker lid and cook on low heat for 8 hours or until the internal temperature of the beef reaches at least 145°F (63°C).

9. Take out the stew from the slow cooker and top with parsley before serving.

Nutrition: **Calories:** 462 - **Total fat:** 34.1g - **Fiber:** 3.2g

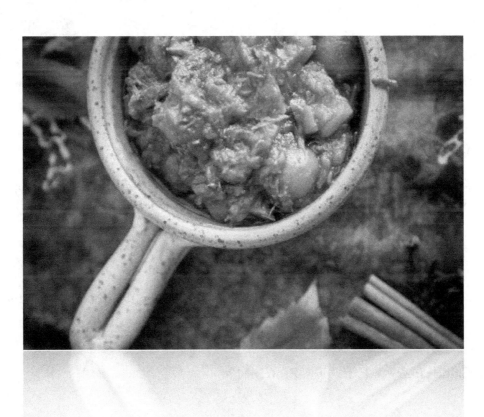

Brussels Sprouts Casserole

Gluten Free, Nut Free

Preparation Time: 15 minutes

Cooking Time: 30 minutes

Servings: 8

Ingredients:

- 8 bacon slices

- 1-pound of Brussels sprouts (blanched for 10 minutes and cut into quarters)

- 1 cup of shredded Swiss cheese (divided)

- ¾ cup of heavy (whipping) cream

Kitchen Equipment:

- oven

- skillet

- casserole dish

- medium bowl

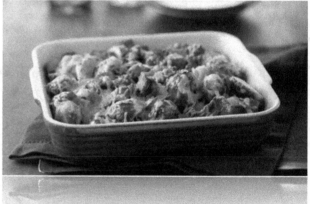

Directions:

1. Set the oven to 400°F. Situate a skillet over medium-high heat and cook the bacon until it is crispy, about 6 minutes.

2. Set aside 1 tablespoon of bacon fat to grease the casserole dish and roughly chop the cooked bacon. Lightly oil a casserole dish with the reserved bacon fat and set aside.

3. In a medium bowl, toss the Brussels sprouts with the chopped bacon and ½ cup of cheese and transfer the mixture to the casserole dish.

4. Transfer the heavy cream over the Brussels sprouts and top the casserole with the remaining ½ cup of cheese. Bake until the cheese is melted and lightly browned and the vegetables are heated through, about 20 minutes. Serve.

Nutrition: **Calories:** 299 - **Fat:** 11g - **Protein:** 12g

Cheesy Mashed Cauliflower

Gluten Free, Nut Free, Vegetarian

Preparation Time: 15 minutes

Cooking Time: 5 minutes

Servings: 4

Ingredients:

- 1 head of cauliflower (chopped roughly)

- ½ cup of shredded cheddar cheese

- ¼ cup of heavy (whipping) cream

- 2 tablespoons of butter (at room temperature)

- Sea salt

- Freshly ground black pepper

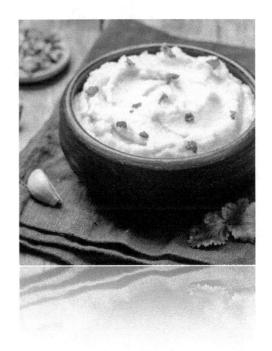

Kitchen Equipment:

- large saucepan

- food processor

Directions:

1. Situate a large saucepan filled three-quarters full with water over high heat and bring to a boil.

2. Blanch the cauliflower until tender, about 5 minutes, and drain.

3. Place the cauliflower to a food processor and add the cheese, heavy cream, and butter.

4. Purée until very creamy and whipped.

5. Season with salt and pepper. Serve.

Nutrition: Calories: 183 - **Fat:** 15g - **Protein** 8g

Mushrooms with Camembert

Gluten Free, Nut Free, Vegetarian

Preparation Time: 5 minutes

Cooking Time: 15 minutes

Servings: 4

Ingredients:

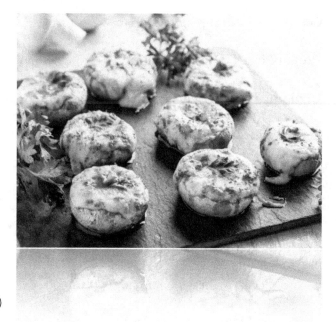

- 2 tablespoons of butter

- 2 teaspoons of minced garlic

- 1-pound of button mushrooms (halved)

- 4 ounces of Camembert cheese (diced)

- Freshly ground black pepper

Kitchen Equipment:

- large skillet

Directions:

1. Situate a large skillet over medium-high heat and melt the butter.

2. Sauté the garlic until translucent, about 3 minutes.

3. Sauté the mushrooms until tender, about 10 minutes.

4. Stir in the cheese and sauté until melted, about 2 minutes.

5. Season with pepper and serve.

Nutrition:

Calories: 161 - **Fat:** 13g - **Protein:** 9g

Vegan Keto Scramble

Preparation Time: 10 minutes

Cooking Time: 15 minutes

Servings: 1

Ingredients:

- 14 oz. of firm tofu

- 3 tbsp. of avocado oil

- 2 tbsp. of yellow onion (diced)

- 1.5 tbsp. of Nutritional yeast

- ½ tsp. of turmeric

- ½ tsp. of garlic powder

- ½ tsp. of salt

- 1 cup of baby spinach

- 3 grape tomatoes

- 3 oz. of vegan cheddar cheese

Kitchen Equipment:

- skillet

Directions:

1. Start by squeezing the water out of the tofu block using a clean cloth or a paper towel.

2. Grab a skillet and put it on medium heat.

3. Sauté the chopped onion in a small amount of avocado oil until it starts to caramelize.

4. Using a potato masher, crumble the tofu on the skillet. Do this thoroughly until the tofu looks a lot like scrambled eggs.

5. Drizzle some more of the avocado oil onto the mix together with the dry seasonings.

6. Stir thoroughly and evenly distribute the flavor.

7. Cook under medium heat, occasionally stirring to avoid burning of the tofu. You'd want most of the liquid to evaporate until you get a nice chunk of scrambled tofu.

8. Fold the baby spinach, cheese, and diced tomato.

9. Cook until the cheese melted.

10. Serve and enjoy!

Nutrition:

Calories: 212 - **Fat:** 17.5g - **Protein:** 10g

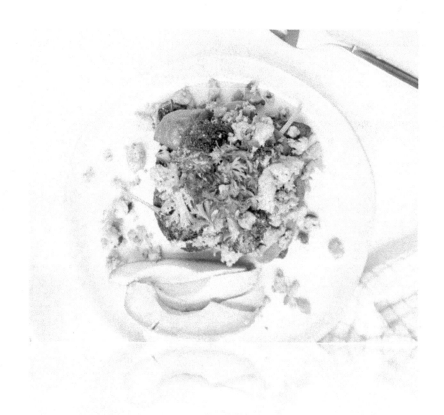

Choco Mousse

Preparation Time: 1 hour

Cooking Time: 0 minute

Servings: 2

Ingredients:

- 4 tbsp. of butter

- 4 tbsp. of cream cheese

- 1 ½ tbsp. of heavy whipping cream

- 1 tbsp. of swerve or another natural sweetener

- 1 tbsp. of unsweetened cocoa powder

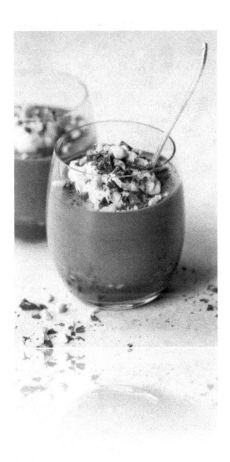

Kitchen Equipment:

- hand mixer

- rubber scraper

Directions:

1. Remove the butter and cream cheese from the fridge for about 30 minutes before time to prepare to become room temperature.

2. Chill a bowl and whisk the cream.

3. Place back in the refrigerator for now.

4. Use a hand mixer to combine the sweetener, cream cheese, cocoa powder, and butter until well mixed.

5. Remove the refrigerated cream and fold it into the chocolate mixture using a rubber scraper.

6. Portion it into two dessert bowls and chill for 1 hour.

Nutrition: Protein: 4g - **Total Fats:** 50g - **Calories** 460

Raspberry Chia Pudding

Preparation Time: 10 minutes

Cooking Time: 0 minute

Servings: 2

Ingredients:

- 4 tbsp. of chia seeds

- ½ cup of raspberries

- 1 cup of coconut milk

Kitchen Equipment:

- 2 mason jars

- blender

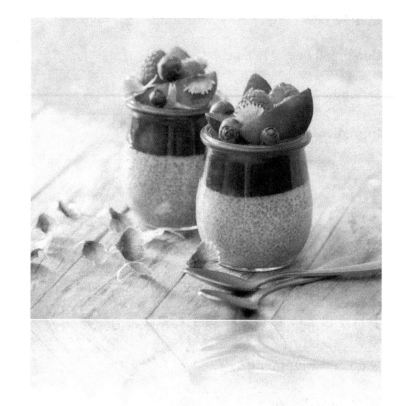

Directions:

1. Pour the milk and raspberries into a blender.

2. Pulse until smooth.

3. Pour into the jars.

4. Fold in the chia seeds and stir.

5. Secure the lid and shake.

6. Store in the fridge for at least three hours before serving.

Nutrition:

Protein: 38.8 - **Total Fats:** 28.3g - **Calories:** 408

Almond Blackberry Chia Pudding

Preparation Time: 15 minutes

Cooking Time: 0 minute

Servings: 2

Ingredients:

- ¼ cup of chia seeds

- Drizzle raw honey

- 2 tbsp. of sliced almonds

- 1 ½ cup of vanilla almond milk

- 6 oz. of fresh blackberries

Kitchen Equipment:

- mixing bowl

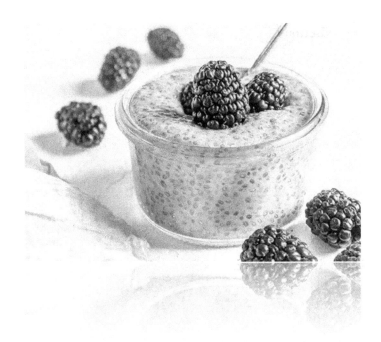

Directions:

1. Rinse and add the berries into a dish.

2. Crush with a fork until creamy.

3. Pour in the raw honey, milk, and chia seeds. Stir well.

4. Let it chill for several hours or overnight for the most delicious results.

5. Sprinkle with the almonds and several blackberries.

6. Serve any time.

Nutrition:

Net Carbohydrates: 1g - **Protein:** 2g - **Calories:** 109

Crunchy Berry Mousse

Preparation Time: 20 minutes

Cooking Time: 0 minute

Servings: 8

Ingredients:

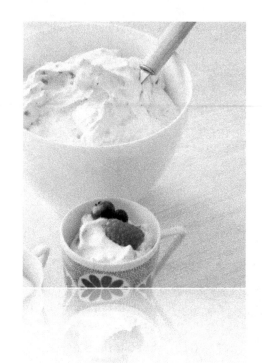

- 2 cups of heavy whipping cream

- ¼ tsp. of vanilla extract

- Lemon zest

- 2 oz. of chopped pecans

- 3 oz. of fresh raspberries/blueberries/strawberries

Kitchen Equipment:

- hand mixer

- plastic wrap

Directions:

1. Use a hand mixer to beat the cream until it forms soft peaks.

2. Then, add the vanilla and lemon zest.

3. Fold in the nuts and berries. Stir.

4. Cover with a layer of plastic wrap.

5. For a firmer mousse, store in the fridge for about 4 hours.

6. You can enjoy it when freshly prepared if you like it less firm.

Nutrition: Protein: 3g - **Total Fats:** 27g - **Calories:** 260

Creme Brulee

Preparation Time: 10 minutes

Cooking Time: 34 minutes

Servings: 4

Ingredients:

- 5 tbsp. of separated natural sweetener (low calorie)
- 4 egg yolks
- 2 cups of heavy whipping cream
- 1 tsp. of vanilla extract

Kitchen Equipment:

- oven
- saucepan
- baking dish

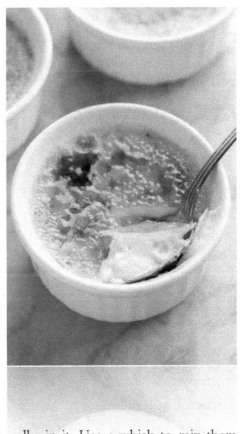

Directions:

1. Preheat the stove at 325 degrees F.
2. Also, get a bowl and put the vanilla extract and egg yolks in it. Use a whisk to mix them properly.
3. Set your stove to medium heat and put a saucepan on it.
4. Add 1 tbsp. of natural sweetener and heavy cream to the pan and mix using a whisk.
5. When you notice the mixture begins to simmer, take the pan down.
6. Get 4 ramekins and separate the mixture equally between them.
7. Place the ramekins in a glass baking dish and add hot water. The water should be 1 inch to the sides of the ramekins.
8. Place the glass baking dish at the center of the oven, and leave it there for 30 minutes. By this time, the Creme Brulee should have set.
9. Add 1 tbsp. of natural sweetener on top of the Creme Brulee.
10. Here's the really cool part: get a culinary torch and flame the sweetener until it turns a golden color and melts.

Nutrition: Calories: 466 - **Carbs:** 16.9g - **Protein:** 5.1g

Keto No-Churn Blueberry Maple Ice Cream

Preparation Time: 10 minutes

Cooking Time: 0 minute

Servings: 3

Ingredients:

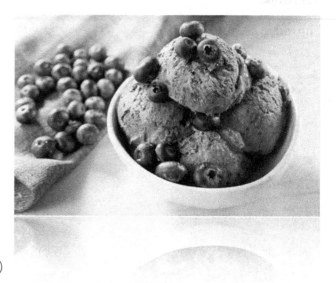

- Pinch of salt

- 1 cup of heavy whipping cream

- ¼ tsp. of xanthan gum

- 1/3 10 oz. of pack blueberries frozen

- ½ tsp. of maple extract

- 2 tbsp. of natural sweetener (low calorie)

- 1 tbsp. of vodka

Kitchen Equipment:

- wide-opening jar

- immersion blender

Directions:

1. Grab a jar that is roughly the same size as a pint and has a wide opening. Put heavy cream, salt, blueberries, xanthan gum, natural sweetener, maple extract, and vodka in it. Process this mixture for about 75 seconds.

2. With an immersion blender, use the up-down motion.

3. The creamy mixture should get considerably thicker by this point.

4. Cover the wide-mouthed jar and pop it in the freezer.

5. In intervals of 35 minutes, stir the cream until it reaches a consistency that you are satisfied with. This might take as much as 4 hours.

Nutrition: Calories: 304 - **Protein:** 1.8g - **Fat:** 29.6g

Gluten Free Bagels

Preparation Time: 15 minutes

Cooking Time: 15 minutes

Servings: 6

Ingredients:

- 2 eggs

- 1 ½ cups of almond flour

- 2 oz. of cubed cream cheese

- 1 tbsp. of baking powder (gluten free)

- 2 ½ cups of mozzarella cheese (shredded)

- 1 tsp. of garlic salt

Kitchen Equipment:

- oven

- baking sheet

- parchment paper

- bowl

- microwave

Directions:

1. Ensure that your oven is heated to 400 degrees F. Also, prepare a baking sheet by lining it with parchment paper.

2. Get a bowl and add the salt, almond flour, and baking powder into it.

3. In a separate bowl that can safely be used in a microwave, add both mozzarella and cream cheese and mix them.

4. Place the bowl containing the cheeses into your microwave and heat for a minute.

5. Take the bowl out, stir the cheeses properly and return it to the microwave.

6. Break the eggs into the bowl and add the baking powder mixture.

7. Using your hands, knead this new mixture until you are left with dough that is quite sticky. Continue working the dough with your hands till the dough is smooth. This should last about 3 minutes.

8. Separate the dough into 6 portions and roll them into thin, round, long strips.

9. Make the ends of each strip of dough connect. It should resemble a bagel now. You are almost done.

10. Place these bagels on the baking sheet you had prepared and bake for about 13 minutes.

11. When the bagels turn an inviting golden-brown color, they are ready to be devoured.

Nutrition:

Calories: 364 - **Protein:** 20.9g - **Fat:** 27.9g

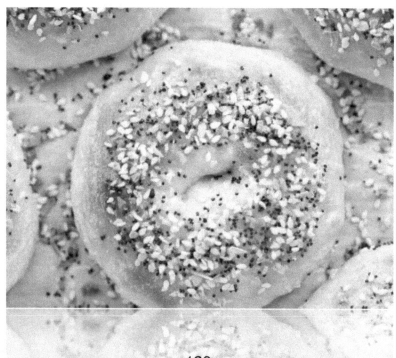

Chapter 6. Recipes from Spain

Avocado Pesto Pasta

Preparation Time: 5 minutes

Cooking Time: 10 minutes

Servings: 2

Ingredients:

- 4 oz. of boneless chicken thighs
- 2 zucchinis
- 4 tbsp. of extra-virgin olive oil
- 1 tbsp. of coconut oil
- 1 avocado
- 1/2 cup of water
- 1/2 cup of fresh basil
- 1 clove of minced garlic
- Salt and pepper to taste

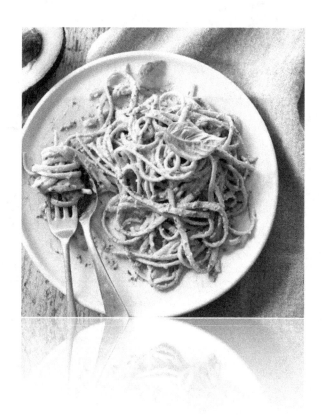

Kitchen Equipment:

- nonstick pan
- spiralizer
- blender

Directions:

1. Heat the coconut oil in a non-stick pan over medium heat.
2. Add the chicken after the oil has melted and cook until the chicken is no longer pink in color.
3. Use a spiralizer while the chicken is cooking and make zoodles out of the zucchinis.
4. Add these to a non-stick pan and cook for around five minutes.
5. Incorporate all other ingredients together in a blender until the mixture is smooth.
6. Add everything to a bowl once the chicken is done.

7. Mix them well so that the avocado sauce we made covers the entire zucchini noodles.

8. Serve them warm and enjoy a scrumptious one!

Nutrition: Calories: 440 - Fat: 40g - Carbohydrates: 16g

Creamy Garlic Chicken

Preparation Time: 5 minutes

Cooking Time: 15 minutes

Servings: 4

Ingredients:

- 4 chicken breasts (finely sliced)
- 1 tsp. of garlic powder
- 1 tsp. of paprika
- 2 tbsp. of butter
- 1 tsp. of salt
- 1 cup of heavy cream
- ½ cup of sun-dried tomatoes
- 2 cloves of garlic (minced)
- 1 cup of spinach (chopped)

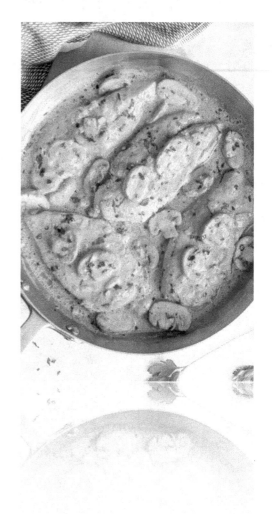

Kitchen Equipment:

- frying pan

Directions:

1. Blend the paprika, garlic powder, and salt and sprinkle over both sides of the chicken.
2. Melt the butter in a frying pan (choose medium heat).
3. Add the chicken breast and fry for 5 minutes each side. Set aside.
4. Add the heavy cream, sun-dried tomatoes, and garlic to the pan and whisk well to combine.
5. Cook for 2 minutes.
6. Add spinach and sauté for an additional 3 minutes.
7. Return the chicken to the pan and cover with the sauce.

Nutrition: Fat: 26g **Protein:** 4g - **Calories** 280

Baked Lemon Salmon

Preparation Time: 10 minutes

Cooking Time: 20 minutes

Servings: 4

Ingredients:

- 4 pcs. of salmon
- A dash salt
- 2 tbsp. of lemon Juice
- 1 lemon
- 2 tbsp. of grass-fed butter
- A dash pepper

Kitchen Equipment:

- stove
- baking sheet
- parchment paper

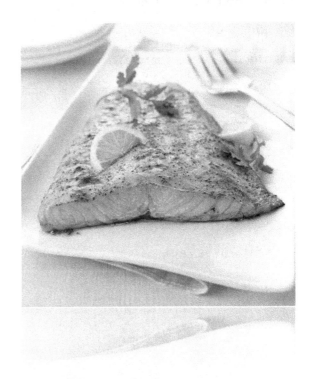

Directions:

1. Preheat the stove to 400°F. As it heats up, get out your baking sheet and line it.

2. When you are set to cook the fish, you will first want to run it under water before patting it down with some paper towels.

3. Once this has been done, place the fish with the skin side facing down.

4. Melt your butter and carefully spoon it over each piece of fish. With the butter in place, you can season with some pepper and salt according to your own taste.

5. Now that the fish has been seasoned, you will then want to pour your lemon juice over the top and place a slice of lemon on top of each salmon filet.

6. When you are ready to cook your meal, you are now going to pop the dish into the stove for fifteen minutes.

7. By the end of this time, you will know that your fish is cooked through if you can flake it easily with a fork. If it is cooked through, take the dish out from the oven and allow it to chill for several minutes.

8. Finally, serve the fish with your favorite Keto-friendly side, and enjoy your meal.

Nutrition: Fats: 20g - **Carbs:** 3g - **Proteins:** 20g

Cilantro and Lime Creamed Chicken

Preparation Time: 10 minutes

Cooking Time: 30 minutes

Servings: 4

Ingredients:

- 4 pcs. of chicken breast
- 1 tsp. of red pepper flakes
- 1 tbsp. of cilantro
- A dash of salt
- 2 tbsp. of lime juice
- 1 cup of chicken broth
- ¼ cup of onion
- 1 tbsp. of olive oil
- ½ cup of heavy cream
- A dash of pepper

Kitchen Equipment:

- skillet

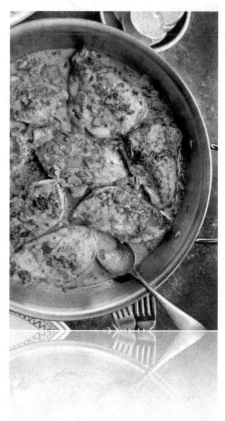

Directions:

1. Get your cooking skillet and place it over a moderate temperature.

2. As the skillet heats, season the chicken breast according to your taste.

3. Once seasoned to your liking, throw the chicken into the skillet and cook for about eight minutes on each side.

4. When the chicken is cooked through, take it out of the pan and place to the side.

5. Stir in the onion into the hot pan and cook them for a minute before also adding in the cilantro, pepper flakes, lime juice, and the chicken broth. If you don't have chicken broth on hand, feel free to use water.

6. Once these items are in place, bring to a boil for 10 minutes.

7. Whisk in your heavy cream and add in the chicken so that it can be coated in the sauce you just made.

8. For extra flavor, add in some more cilantro, and then your chicken can be served by itself or with a Keto-friendly vegetable!

Nutrition: Fats: 20g - **Carbs:** 6g - **Proteins:** 30g

Creamed Spinach

Gluten Free, Nut Free

Preparation Time: 10 minutes

Cooking Time: 30 minutes

Servings: 4

Ingredients:

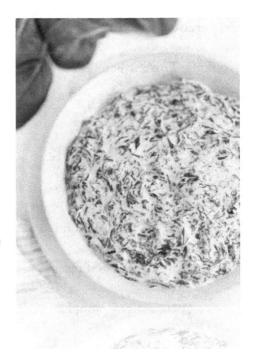

- 1 tablespoon of butter

- ½ sweet onion (very thinly sliced)

- 4 cups of spinach (stemmed and thoroughly washed)

- ¾ cup of heavy (whipping) cream

- ¼ cup of herbed chicken stock

- Pinch of sea salt

- Pinch of freshly ground black pepper

- Pinch of ground nutmeg

Kitchen Equipment:

- large skillet

Directions:

1. Melt butter in a large skillet over medium heat.

2. Sauté the onion until it is lightly caramelized, about 5 minutes.

3. Stir in the spinach, heavy cream, chicken stock, salt, pepper, and nutmeg.

4. Sauté until the spinach is wilted, about 5 minutes.

5. Continue cooking the spinach until it is tender and the sauce is thickened, about 15 minutes.

6. Serve immediately.

Nutrition: Calories: 195 - **Fat:** 20g - **Protein** 3g

Nut Medley Granola

Dairy Free, Gluten Free, Vegetarian

Preparation Time: 10 minutes

Cooking Time: 1 hour

Servings: 8

Ingredients:

- 2 cups of shredded unsweetened coconut

- 1 cup of sliced almonds

- 1 cup of raw sunflower seeds

- ½ cup of raw pumpkin seeds

- ½ cup of walnuts

- ½ cup of melted coconut oil

- 10 drops of liquid stevia

- 1 teaspoon of ground cinnamon

- ½ teaspoon of ground nutmeg

Kitchen Equipment:

- oven

- 2 baking sheets

- parchment paper

- large bowl

- small bowl

Directions:

1. Preheat the oven to 250°F.

2. Line 2 baking sheets with parchment paper. Set aside.

3. Combine together the shredded coconut, almonds, sunflower seeds, pumpkin seeds, and walnuts in a large bowl.

4. In a small bowl, mix together the coconut oil, stevia, cinnamon, and nutmeg.

5. Pour the coconut oil mixture into the nut mixture and use your hands to blend until the nuts are very well coated.

6. Transfer the granola mixture to the baking sheets and spread it out evenly.

7. Bake the granola, stirring every 10 to 15 minutes, until the mixture is golden brown and crunchy, about 1 hour.

8. Transfer the granola to a large bowl and let the granola cool, tossing it frequently to break up the large pieces.

9. Store the granola in airtight containers in the refrigerator or freezer for up to 1 month.

Nutrition:

Calories: 391- **Fat:** 38g - **Protein:** 10g

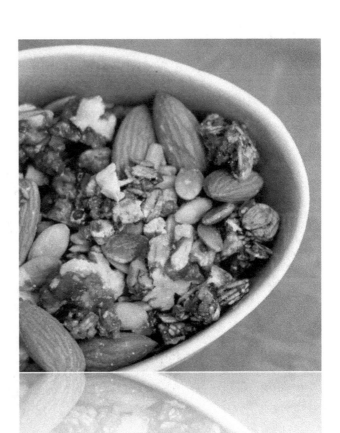

Spicy and Sour Chicken Stew

Preparation Time: 10 minutes

Cooking Time: 80 minutes

Servings: 6

Ingredients:

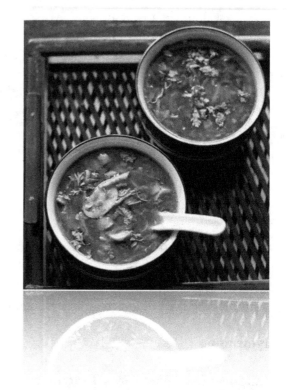

- 2 tablespoons of extra-virgin olive oil
- 6 chicken thighs (skin on, boneless)
- 1 chicken stock cube
- 1 red chili (finely chopped)
- 1 small onion (finely chopped)
- 2 limes
- 2 tins chopped tomatoes
- 3 garlic cloves (crushed)
- Salt and black pepper (to taste)
- 1 cup of water
- Large handful of fresh coriander (chopped)

Kitchen Equipment:

- slow cooker

Directions:

1. Grease the insert of the slow cooker with 2 tablespoons of olive oil.

2. Combine the remaining ingredients, except for the coriander, in the slow cooker.

3. Stir to mix well.

4. Put the slow cooker lid on and cook on low heat for 6 hours.

5. Place the stew to a large bowl.

6. Top it with coriander and slice to serve.

Nutrition: Calories: 445 - **Total fat:** 32.2g - **Fiber:** 1.1g

Sauerkraut and Sausage Soup

Preparation Time: 15 minutes

Cooking Time: 75 minutes

Servings: 6

Ingredients:

- 1 tablespoon of extra-virgin olive oil

- 1 pound (454 g) organic sausage (cooked and sliced)

- 2 cups of sauerkraut

- ½ teaspoon of caraway seeds

- 1 sweet onion (chopped)

- 1 tablespoon of hot mustard

- 2 tablespoons of butter

- 2 celery stalks (chopped)

- 2 teaspoons of minced garlic

- 6 cups of beef broth

- ½ cup of sour cream

- 2 tablespoons of chopped fresh parsley (for garnish)

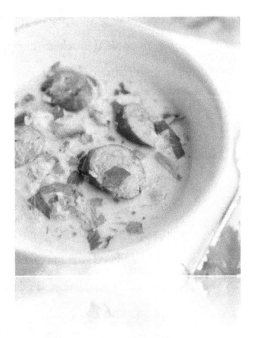

Kitchen Equipment:

- slow cooker

Directions:

1. Grease the insert of the slow cooker with olive oil.

2. Combine the remaining ingredients, except for the sour cream and parsley, in the slow cooker. Stir to mix well.

3. Place the slow cooker lid on and cook on low heat for 6 hours.

4. Put the soup into a large bowl, and mix in the sour cream. Top with parsley and serve warm.

Nutrition: Calories: 333 - **Total fat:** 28.1g - **Fiber:** 2.1g

Jambalaya Broth

Preparation Time: 15 minutes

Cooking Time: 70 minutes

Servings: 8

Ingredients:

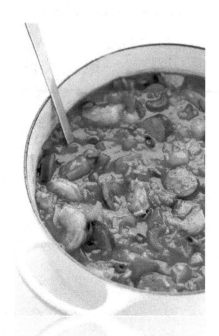

- 1 tablespoon of extra-virgin olive oil
- 6 cups chicken broth
- 1 (28-ounce / 794-g) can of tomatoes (diced)
- 1 pound (454 g) of spicy organic sausage (sliced)
- 1 cup of cooked chicken (chopped)
- 1 red bell pepper (chopped)
- ½ sweet onion (chopped)
- 1 jalapeño pepper (chopped)
- 2 teaspoons of garlic (minced)
- 3 tablespoons of Cajun seasoning
- ½ pound (227 g) of medium shrimp (peeled, deveined, and chopped)
- ½ cup of sour cream (for garnish)
- 1 avocado (diced, for garnish)
- 2 tablespoons of chopped cilantro (for garnish)

Kitchen Equipment:

- slow cooker

Directions:

1. Grease the insert of the slow cooker with olive oil.
2. Combine the chicken, sausage, broth, tomatoes, onion, jalapeño, bell pepper, Cajun seasoning, and garlic in the slow cooker. Stir to mix well.
3. Situate the slow cooker lid on and cook on low heat for 6 hours.
4. Stir in the shrimp and cook for an additional 30 minutes or until the fresh of the shrimp is opaque and a little white in color.
5. Transfer the soup into a large bowl.
6. Add the avocado, sour cream, and cilantro, and then stir to mix well before serving warm.

Nutrition:

Calories: 402 - **Total fat:** 31.1g - **Fiber:** 4.2g

Creamy Cauliflower and Celery Soup with Crisp Bacon

Preparation Time: 5 minutes

Cooking Time: 20 minutes

Servings: 4

Ingredients:

- 2 tablespoons of olive oil
- 1 onion (chopped)
- 1 head of cauliflower (cut into florets)
- ¼ celery root (grated)
- 3 cups of water
- Salt and black pepper (to taste)
- 1 cup of white cheddar cheese (shredded)
- 1 cup of almond milk
- 2 ounces (57 g) of bacon (cut into strips)

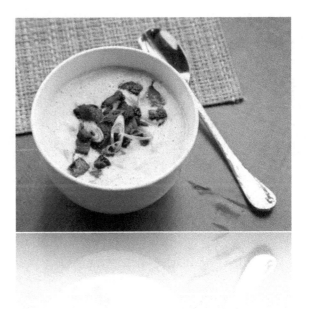

Kitchen Equipment:

- stockpot
- immersion blender
- nonstick skillet
- bowl

Directions:

1. Grease the olive oil in a stockpot over medium heat until shimmering.
2. Add the onion to the pot and sauté for 3 minutes or until translucent.
3. Add the cauliflower florets and celery root to the pot and sauté for 3 minutes or until tender.
4. Pour the water into the pot, and sprinkle salt and black pepper to season.
5. Stir to combine well and bring to a boil.
6. Turn down the heat to low and put the lid on to cook for 10 minutes.
7. Use an immersion blender to mix the ingredients in the soup entirely, and then mix in the cheese and almond milk.
8. Fry the bacon in a nonstick skillet over high heat for 5 minutes or until curls and buckle.
9. Flip the bacon halfway through the cooking time.
10. Divide the soup into four bowls and top with bacon. Serve hot.

Nutrition: - Calories: 365 - **Total fat:** 27.2g - **Protein:** 22.7g

Lamb Curry Stew

Preparation Time: 15 minutes

Cooking Time: 50 minutes

Servings: 4

Ingredients:

- 1 tablespoon of olive oil

- 1 small yellow onion (chopped)

- 1½ pounds (680 g) of boneless lamb shoulder (chopped)

- 1 tablespoon of curry powder

- 1½ cups of chicken broth

- 2 cups of chopped cauliflower

- Salt and black pepper (to taste)

Kitchen Equipment:

- nonstick skillet

- pressure cooker

- large bowl

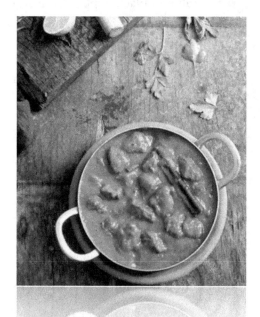

Directions:

1. Heat the olive oil in a nonstick skillet over medium-high heat until shimmering.

2. Add the onion to the skillet and sauté for 4 minutes or until translucent.

3. Add the remaining ingredients and sauté to combine well.

4. Transfer all of them into a pressure cooker.

5. Put the lid on and cook for 50 minutes.

6. Release the pressure, then remove the stew from the pressure cooker to a large bowl and serve warm.

Nutrition: Calories: 386 - **Total fat:** 14.7g - **Fiber:** 2.1g

Smoothie Green Soup

Preparation Time: 5 minutes

Cooking Time: 25 minutes

Servings: 4

Ingredients:

- 2 tablespoons of coconut oil
- ½ cup of leeks
- 1 onion (chopped)
- 1 garlic clove (minced)
- 1 broccoli head (chopped)
- 3 cups of vegetable stock
- 1 bay leaf
- 1 cup of spinach (blanched)
- ½ cup of coconut milk
- Salt and black pepper (to taste)
- 2 tablespoons of coconut yogurt (for garnish)

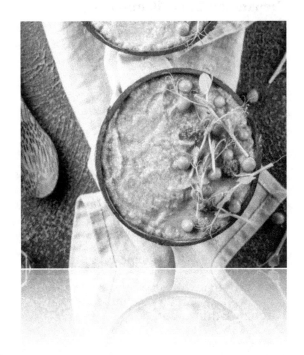

Kitchen Equipment:

- pot
- immersion blender

Directions:

1. Heat the coconut oil in a stockpot over medium heat until shimmering.
2. Add the leeks, onion, and garlic to the pot and cook for 5 minutes or until the onion is translucent.
3. Mix the broccoli to the pot and cook for 5 minutes more or until tender.
4. Pour the vegetable stock in the pot, and add the bay leaf.
5. Put the lid on and bring the soup to a boil.
6. Reduce the heat to low and simmer for 10 minutes.
7. Stir in the spinach to the pot and simmer for 3 minutes.
8. Use an immersion blender to fully mix the soup.
9. Mix in the coconut milk, then season with salt and black pepper.
10. Discard the bay leaf and divide the soup into four bowls, then top with coconut yogurt before serving.

Nutrition:

Calories: 273 - **Total fat:** 24.6g - **Protein:** 4.6g

Sausage Balls

Preparation Time: 10 minutes

Cooking Time: 45 minutes

Servings: 6

Ingredients:

- 1 pound of spicy pork sausage (ground)
- 8 ounces of cream cheese
- 1/2 cup of cheddar cheese (shredded)
- 1/3 cup of parmesan cheese (shredded)
- 1 tbsp. of Dijon mustard
- 1/2 tsp. of garlic powder
- 1/4 tsp. of salt

Kitchen Equipment:

- oven
- parchment paper
- baking sheet

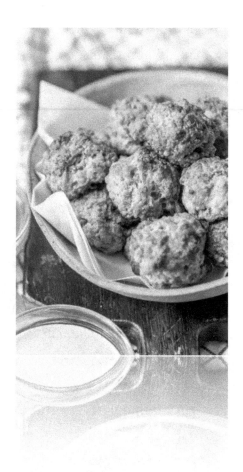

Directions:

1. Preheat your oven at 170 degrees Celsius.
2. Use parchment paper for lining a baking sheet.
3. Combine cream cheese, sausage, parmesan cheese, cheddar cheese, garlic powder, mustard, and salt in a mixing bowl. Mix well.
4. Take 1 tbsp. of the mixture. Roll it into a ball.
5. Repeat for the remaining mixture.
6. Arrange the prepared balls on the lined baking tray.
7. Bake for 30 minutes.
8. Serve hot.

Nutrition:

Calories: 102.3 - **Protein:** 5.9g - **Fat:** 9.6g

Grilled Turkey Burger

Preparation Time: 5 minutes

Cooking Time: 10 minutes

Servings: 4

Ingredients:

- 1 lb. of ground turkey breasts

- 1/2 cup of almond flour

- 1 large egg

- 1/4 cup of yellow onion

- 1/4 cup of chopped parsley

- 1 clove of minced garlic

- 1 tbsp. of extra-virgin olive oil

- Salt and pepper to taste

Kitchen Equipment:

- bowl

- nonstick grilling pan

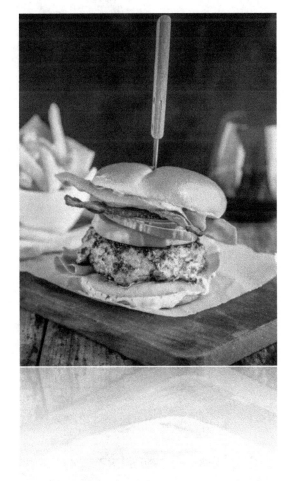

Directions:

1. In a bowl, mix turkey, egg, almond flour, parsley, garlic and onions. Season it, and then mix them all well.

2. Evenly shape the mixture into four identical patties.

3. Use extra-virgin olive oil with brush on both sides.

4. Add some oil to a non-stick grilling pan on medium-high heat.

5. Now, place the patties you made on the grill and cook for about five to six minutes.

6. Turn the patties and cook for another five to six minutes.

7. Finally, wrap the patties in a lettuce and eat away!

Nutrition: Calories: 340 - **Fat:** 21g - **Fiber:** 2.5g

Chipotle Steak with Tortilla

Preparation Time: 5 minutes

Cooking Time: 15 minutes

Servings: 4

Ingredients:

- 16 oz. of skirt steak

- 4 oz. of pepper jack cheese

- 1 cup of sour cream

- 1 handful of fresh cilantro

- 1 tbsp. of extra-virgin olive oil

- 1 splash of chipotle tabasco sauce

- Salt and pepper to taste

- Homemade guacamole

- 2 avocado(s)

- 2 tsp. of lime juice

- 2 tbsp. of fresh cilantro

- Salt and pepper to taste

Kitchen Equipment:

- cast iron skillet

Directions:

1. Season your skirt steak to taste with salt and pepper.

2. Then, on high heat, heat a cast iron skillet.

3. Pour olive oil when the skillet is hot and cook the skirt steak for around four minutes on each side.

4. Transfer it on a plate to rest while you prepare the guacamole.

5. Slice the steak against the grain and make it into bite-sized strips.

6. Divide the same into four equal portions.

7. Add the cheese to the top portion.

8. Follow that with ¼ cup of guacamole and ¼ cup of sour cream.

9. Splash each portion with some chipotle tabasco sauce (not necessary) and fresh cilantro.

10. Prepare the guacamole and serve with low carb tortillas.

11. For homemade guacamole, remove the pit from the avocado and then mash the content.

12. Add the rest of the ingredients and serve.

Nutrition:

Calories: 810 - **Fat:** 61g - **Carbohydrates:** 15g

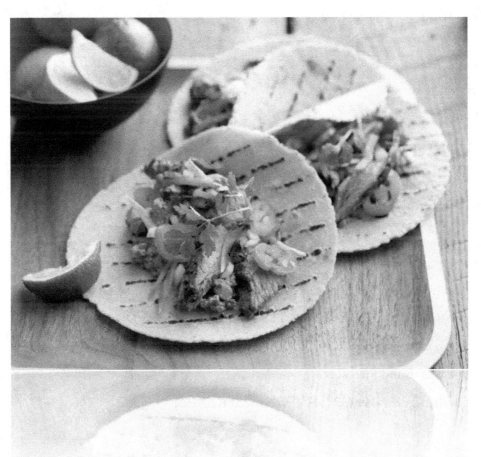

Chicken Avocado Egg Bacon

Preparation Time: 10 minutes

Cooking Time: 10 minutes

Servings: 4

Ingredients:

- 12 oz. of cooked chicken breast
- 6 slices of crumbled bacon
- 3 boiled eggs cut into cubes
- 1 cup of cherry tomatoes cut into halves
- 1/2 small sliced red onion
- 1 large avocado
- 1/2 stick finely chopped of celery
- Salad dressing
- 1/2 cup of olive oil mayonnaise
- 2 tbsp. of sour cream
- 1 tsp. of Dijon mustard
- 4 tbsp. of extra-virgin olive oil
- 2 cloves of minced garlic
- 2 tsp. of lemon juice
- 4 cups of lettuce
- Salt and pepper to taste

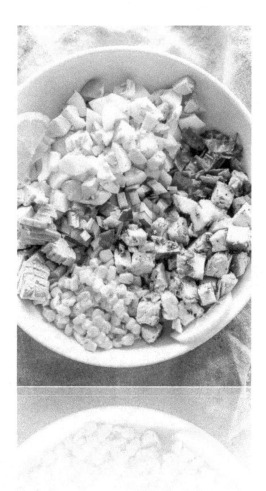

Kitchen Equipment:

- Bowl

Directions:

1. Mix well all the ingredients together for the salad dressing.
2. Then, combine chicken, tomatoes, bacon, eggs, red onions, and celery together.
3. Add about ¾ of the salad dressing and mix them well.
4. Add the avocado and toss together gently.
5. Check the taste and, if needed, add the remainder of the salad dressing as well.
6. Season to taste and then serve it over lettuce.

Nutrition: Calories: 387 - **Fat:** 27g - **Carbohydrates:** 2.5g

Bacon Wrapped Chicken Breast

Preparation Time: 10 minutes

Cooking Time: 45 minutes

Servings: 4

Ingredients:

- 4 boneless (skinless chicken breasts)

- 8 oz. of sharp cheddar cheese

- 8 slices of bacon

- 4 oz. of sliced jalapeño peppers

- 1 tsp. of garlic powder

- Salt and pepper to taste

Kitchen Equipment:

- oven

- nonstick baking sheet

- broiler

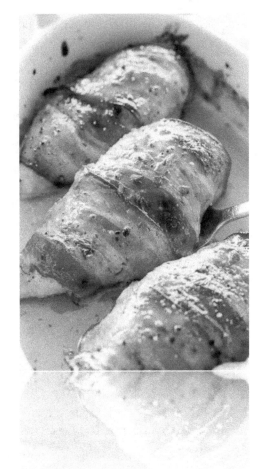

Directions:

1. Preheat the oven at around 350°F.

2. Ensure to season both sides of chicken breast well with salt, garlic powder, and pepper.

3. Place the chicken breast on a non-stick baking sheet (foil-covered).

4. Cover the chicken with cheese and add jalapeño slices.

5. Cut the bacon slices in half and then place the four halves over each piece of chicken.

6. Bake for around 30 to 45 minutes at most. If the chicken is set but the bacon still feels undercooked, you may need to situate it under the broiler for few minutes.

7. Once done, serve hot with a side of low carb garlic parmesan roasted asparagus.

Nutrition:Calories: 640 **Fat:** 48g - **Carbohydrates** 6g

Low Carb Ramen

Preparation Time: 10 minutes

Cooking Time: 30 minutes

Servings: 4

Ingredients:

- 4 cups of filtered water
- 4 pastured eggs
- 1 tbsp. of sugar-free red curry paste
- 1 tbsp. of coconut oil
- 2 tsp. of ground ginger
- 1 tsp. of ground turmeric
- 1 tsp. of garlic powder
- 2 cups of full-fat canned coconut milk
- 1 cup of purple cabbage (chopped)
- 1 cup of large-sized shredded rainbow carrots
- 1 cup of Brussels sprouts (halved)
- 2 large zucchinis (spiralized)
- Salt and pepper to taste

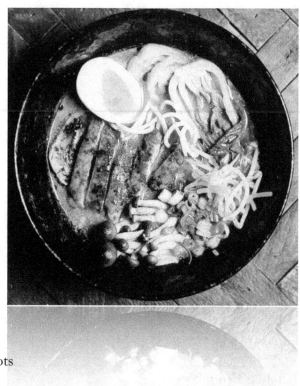

Kitchen Equipment:

- large pot

Directions:

1. Grab a large pot and pour the water inside it, bringing it to a boil.
2. When boiling, add the coconut milk and spices.
3. Reduce the heat to medium-low. Put in the cabbage, Brussels sprouts, and carrots.
4. Stir in a while before adding the curry paste and coconut oil.
5. Continue cooking until the vegetables are soft and tender. This should take about 20 minutes.
6. While waiting, soft boil the eggs. This should take about 6 minutes.
7. Take it out of the pot and put in cold water.
8. When the vegetables are soft, put in the zucchini and allow it to cook for 4 minutes. Your vegetarian ramen is ready.
9. Serve it with the peeled and halved eggs.
10. Put in some lime juice and cilantro.

Nutrition: Calories: 237 - **Fat:** 15g - **Total carbohydrates:** 15g

Low Carb Smoked Salmon Chowder

Preparation Time: 10 minutes

Cooking Time: 20 minutes

Servings: 6

Ingredients:

- 1 stalk celery (chopped)
- 1 clove of garlic (minced)
- 2 tbsp. of salted butter
- 2 tbsp. of capers
- 2 tbsp. of chopped red onion
- 1 tbsp. of tomato paste
- ½ tsp. of salt
- ¼ cup of chopped onion
- 1½ cups of chicken broth
- 1½ cups of heavy whipping cream
- 4 oz. of cream cheese
- 6 oz. of smoked salmon hot smoked (chopped)

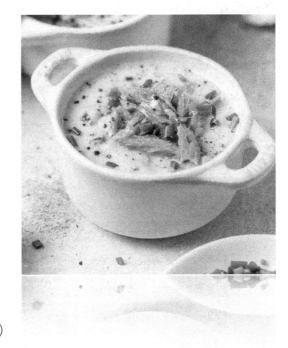

Kitchen Equipment:

- large saucepan
- blender

Directions:

1. Grab a large saucepan and melt butter in it using medium heat.
2. Put onion, celery, and sprinkle some salt onto the pan.
3. Sauté until the vegetables are tender.
4. Put in the onion until fragrant.
5. Add the chicken broth and tomato paste.
6. Allow the mix to simmer, constantly stirring until you get a smooth concoction.
7. In the meantime, transfer the cream cheese in a blender and put some of the broth mixture inside it.
8. Blend until smooth. You can do this slowly if this will make it easier.
9. Put the broth back in the saucepan and add the salmon, capers, and cream.
10. Allow it to simmer again for a few minutes.
11. The soup is ready now. Before serving, try sprinkling some chopped red onion on top.

Nutrition:

Calories: 373

Carbohydrates: 31.84g

Fiber: 0.5g

Slow Cooker Vegetable Beef

Preparation Time: 10 minutes

Cooking Time: 70 minutes

Servings: 12

Ingredients:

- 4 slices of bacon (sliced into 1/2-inch pieces)
- 2 pounds of stew meat (cut into 1" cubes)
- 1 small celeriac (diced)
- 2 tbsp. of red wine vinegar
- 2 tbsp. of tomato paste
- 1/2 tsp. of dried rosemary
- 1/2 tsp. of dried thyme
- 1/2 tsp. of ground black pepper
- 1 tsp. of sea salt
- 1/4 cup of green beans (cut into 1-inch pieces)
- 1/4 cup of carrots (diced)
- 1 28 oz. can of diced tomatoes
- 2 cloves of garlic (crushed)
- 32 oz. of beef broth low-sodium
- 1 medium yellow onion (chopped)

Kitchen Equipment:

- large skillet
- slow cooker

Directions:

1. Situate a large skillet on medium high heat. Cook the bacon until crispy and store it in the fridge for later.

2. Remove most of the bacon grease, keeping only a small amount enough to cook the beef cubes in small batches. Season them with salt and pepper.

3. Cook until the beef cubes are browned. No need to cook the meat thoroughly, just sear it a little at the side.

4. When brown, place the beef in a slow cooker crock.

5. Once all the beef cubes are in the slow cooker, turn your attention to the skillet.

6. Lower the heat to medium and add vinegar to the skillet.

7. Stir the vinegar around until you get a thicker consistency.

8. Pour ¼ cup of the broth in the skillet. When done, pour the liquid in the slow cooker.

9. Remember, we only transferred ¼ cup of the broth to the skillet. The remaining broth will now be cooked in the pan. This time, you'll beading the celeriac, carrots, diced tomatoes, tomato paste, onion, green beans, rosemary, thyme, and salt to the mixture.

10. Put some pepper as well depending on the taste.

11. Cook for 5 minutes before transferring the whole thin to the slow cooker as well. Stir constantly for 5 minutes.

12. Cover the slow cooker and set it to run for 7 hours. Taste every 2 hours and adjust as needed. Garnish with the bacon bits when serving.

Nutrition:

Calories: 212 - **Fat:** 13g - **Carbohydrates:** 6g

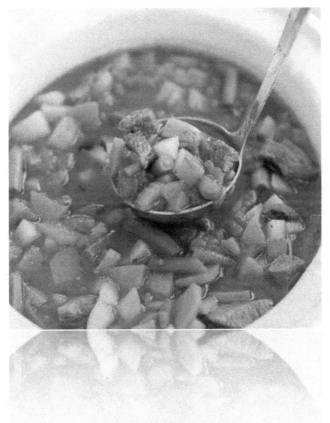

Keto Chicken

Preparation Time: 10 minutes

Cooking Time: 40 minutes

Servings: 4

Ingredients:

- 2 tbsp. of avocado oil
- 2 stalks celery (chopped)
- 4 cups of chicken broth
- 2 cups of riced cauliflower
- 1/2 tsp. of dried thyme leaves
- 1/2 tsp. of paprika
- 1/4 cup of chopped onions
- 2 cloves of garlic (minced)
- 1 lb. of skinless (boneless chicken thighs)
- salt and pepper (to taste)

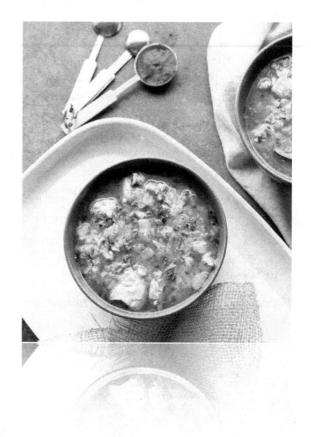

Kitchen Equipment:

- large saucepan

Directions:

1. Start by grabbing a large saucepan and heating the oil over medium heat.
2. Put in the onion and celery. Season it with salt and pepper before cooking.
3. Wait until the vegetable becomes soft before adding the garlic, paprika, and thyme. You should be able to get a fragrant smell
4. Put in the broth and stir for a few minutes.
5. Add the rice cauliflower and the chicken.
6. Allow it to boil before reducing it to simmer. This should take about 12 minutes or until the chicken is cooked all the way to the center.
7. Add salt and pepper to taste.

Nutrition: Calories: 196 - **Fat:** 10.4g - **Fiber:** 1.8g

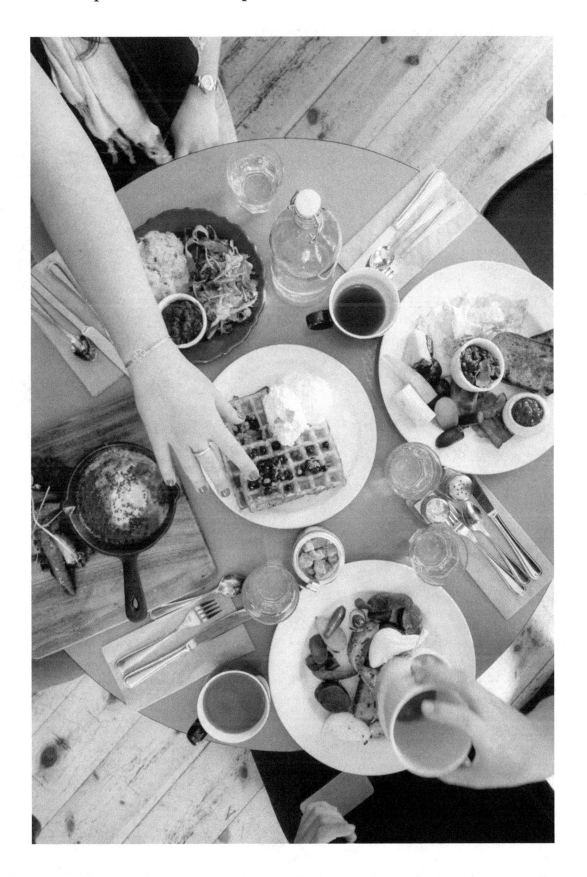

Pork Cutlets with Spanish Onion

Preparation Time: 15 minutes

Cooking Time: 15 minutes

Servings: 4

Ingredients:

- 1 tablespoon of olive oil

- 2 pork cutlets

- 1 bell pepper (deveined and sliced)

- 1 Spanish of onion (chopped)

- 2 garlic cloves (minced)

- 1/2 teaspoon of hot sauce

- 1/2 teaspoon of mustard

- 1/2 teaspoon of paprika

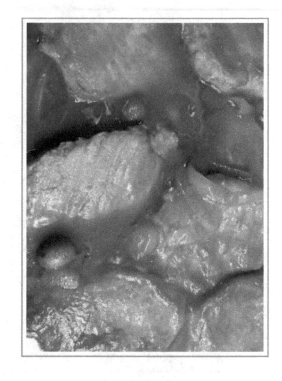

Kitchen Equipment:

- saucepan

Directions:

1. Fry the pork cutlets for 3 to 4 minutes until evenly golden and crispy on both sides.

2. Set the temperature to medium and add the bell pepper, Spanish onion, garlic, hot sauce, and mustard; continue cooking until the vegetables have softened, for a further 3 minutes.

3. Sprinkle with paprika, salt, and black pepper.

4. Serve immediately and enjoy!

Nutrition: Calories: 403 - **Fat:** 24.1g - **Total Carbs:** 3.4g

Rich and Easy Pork Ragout

Preparation Time: 15 minutes

Cooking Time: 15 minutes

Servings: 4

Ingredients:

- 1 teaspoon of lard (melted at room temperature)
- 3/4-pound of pork butt (cut into bite-sized cubes)
- 1 red bell pepper (deveined and chopped)
- 1 poblano pepper (deveined and chopped)
- 2 cloves of garlic (pressed)
- 1/2 cup of leeks, chopped
- 1/2 teaspoon of mustard seeds
- 1/4 teaspoon of ground allspice
- 1/4 teaspoon of celery seeds
- 1 cup of roasted vegetable broth
- 2 vine-ripe tomatoes (pureed)

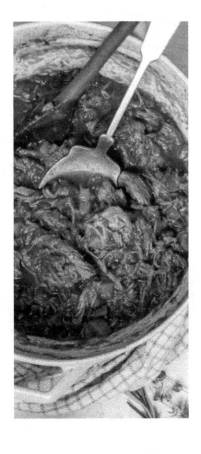

Kitchen Equipment:

- stockpot

Directions:

1. Melt the lard in a stockpot over moderate heat.

2. Once hot, cook the pork cubes for 4 to 6 minutes, occasionally stirring to ensure even cooking.

3. Then, stir in the vegetables and continue cooking until they are tender and fragrant.

4. Add in the salt, black pepper, mustard seeds, allspice, celery seeds, roasted vegetable broth, and tomatoes.

5. Reduce the heat to simmer. Let it simmer for 30 minutes longer or until everything is heated through.

6. Ladle into individual bowls and serve hot. Bon appétit!

Nutrition: Calories: 389 - **Fat:** 24.3g - **Total Carbs:** 5.4g

Melt-in-Your-Mouth Pork Roast

Preparation Time: 35 minutes

Cooking Time: 40 minutes

Servings: 2

Ingredients:

1-pound pork shoulder

4 tablespoons red wine

1 teaspoon stone-ground mustard

1 tablespoon coconut aminos

1 tablespoon lemon juice

1 tablespoon sesame oil

2 sprigs rosemary

1 teaspoon sage

1shallot, peeled and chopped

1/2 celery stalk, chopped

1/2 head garlic, separated into cloves

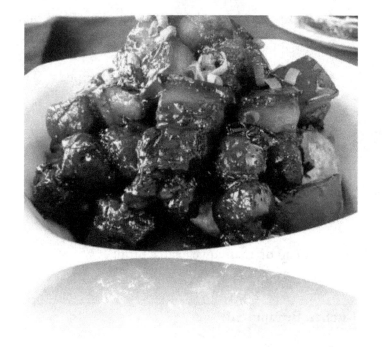

Kitchen Equipment:

ceramic dish

baking dish

Directions:

Place the pork shoulder, red wine, mustard, coconut aminos, lemon juice, sesame oil, rosemary, and sage in a ceramic dish; cover and let it marinate in your refrigerator at least 1 hour.

Discard a lightly greased baking dish. Scatter the vegetables around the pork shoulder and sprinkle with salt and black pepper. Roast in the preheated oven at 390 degrees F for 15 minutes.

Now, reduce the temperature to 310 degrees F and continue baking an additional 40 to 45 minutes. Baste the meat with the reserved marinade once or twice.

Place on cooling racks before carving and serving. Bon appétit!

Nutrition: Calories 497 - **Fat** 35g - **Protein** 40.2g

Chunky Pork Soup with Mustard Greens

Preparation Time: 25 minutes

Cooking Time: 30 minutes

Servings: 2

Ingredients:

1tablespoon olive oil

1 bell pepper, deveined and chopped

2 garlic cloves, pressed

1/2 cup scallions, chopped

1/2-pound ground pork (84% lean)

1 cup beef bone broth

1 cup of water

1/2 teaspoon crushed red pepper flakes

1 bay laurel

1 teaspoon fish sauce

2 cups mustard greens, torn into pieces

1 tablespoon fresh parsley, chopped

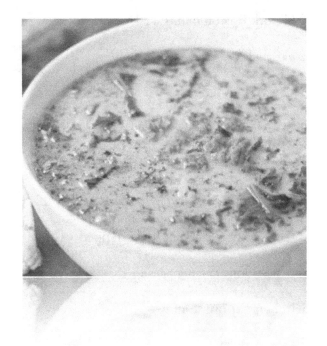

Kitchen Equipment:

sauté pan

Directions:

Coat, once hot, sauté the pepper, garlic, and scallions until tender or about 3 minutes.

After that, stir in the ground pork and cook for 5 minutes more or until well browned, stirring periodically.

Add in the beef bone broth, water, red pepper, salt, black pepper, and bay laurel. Reduce the temperature to simmer and cook, covered, for 10 minutes. Afterward, stir in the fish sauce and mustard greens.

Remove from the heat; let it stand until the greens are wilted. Ladle into individual bowls and serve garnished with fresh parsley.

Nutrition: Calories 344 - **Fat** 25.g

Pulled Pork with Mint and Cheese

Preparation Time: 20 minutes

Cooking Time: 15 minutes

Servings: 2

Ingredients:

1 teaspoon lard, melted at room temperature

3/4 pork Boston butt, sliced

2 garlic cloves, pressed

1/2 teaspoon red pepper flakes, crushed

1/2 teaspoon black peppercorns, freshly cracked

Sea salt, to taste

2 bell peppers, deveined and sliced

1 tablespoon fresh mint leave snipped

4 tablespoons cream cheese

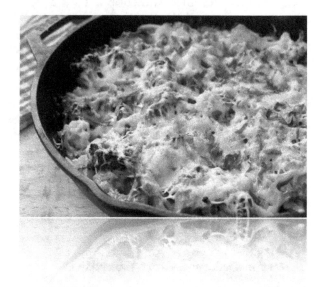

Kitchen Equipment:

cast-iron skillet

Directions:

Melt the lard in a cast-iron skillet over a moderate flame. Once hot, brown the pork for 2 minutes per side until caramelized and crispy on the edges.

Set the temperature to medium-low and continue cooking another 4 minutes, turning over periodically. Shred the pork with two forks and return to the skillet.

Add the garlic, red pepper, black peppercorns, salt, and bell pepper and continue cooking for a further 2 minutes or until the peppers are just tender and fragrant.

Serve with fresh mint and a dollop of cream cheese. Enjoy!

Nutrition: Calories 370 - **Fat** 21.9g - **Protein:** 34.9g

Pork Loin Steaks in Creamy Pepper Sauce

Preparation Time: 15 minutes

Cooking Time: 10 minutes

Servings: 2

Ingredients:

1 teaspoon lard, at room temperature

2 pork loin steaks

1/2 cup beef bone broth

2 bell peppers, deseeded and chopped

1 shallot, chopped

1 garlic clove, minced

Sea salt, to season

1/2 teaspoon cayenne pepper

1/4 teaspoon paprika

1 teaspoon Italian seasoning mix

1/4 cup Greek-style yogurt

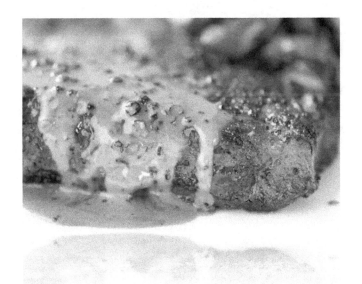

Kitchen Equipment:

cast-iron skillet

Directions:

Melt the lard in a cast-iron skillet over moderate heat. Once hot, cook the pork loin steaks until slightly browned or approximately 5 minutes per side; reserve.

Add a splash of the beef bone broth to deglaze the pan. Now, cook the bell peppers, shallot, and garlic until tender and aromatic—season with salt, cayenne pepper, paprika, and Italian seasoning mix.

After that, decrease the temperature to medium-low, add the Greek yogurt to the skillet and let it simmer for 2 minutes more or until heated through. Serve immediately.

Nutrition: Calories 447 - **Fat**19.2g - **Protein:** 62.2g

Another Low Carb Keto Chicken

Preparation Time: 10 minutes

Cooking Time: 30 minutes

Servings: 4

Ingredients:

- 1 1/4 small yellow onion

- 2 medium carrots (peeled and chopped)

- 1 small leek (chopped)

- 3 medium stalks celery (chopped)

- liters chicken stock

- 1 cup of chopped kale

- 1/4 tsp. of black pepper

- 1 tbsp. of butter

- 1 tbsp. of thyme leaves chopped

- 300g of cooked chicken

- 2 bay leaves

- 8g of fresh parsley

- 1 garlic clove minced

- Salt to taste

- Squeeze of lemon juice (for serving)

- 1 tbsp. of olive oil (for serving)

- 1 tsp. of fresh parsley (for serving)

Kitchen Equipment:

- pot

- stick blender

Directions:

1. Grab a soup pot and put 1 tablespoon of butter or olive oil.

2. Cook it over medium heat and sauté the onion, celery, leek, carrots, and thyme in the pan. Wait until they start to soften.

3. Put in the stock and bay leaves.

4. Season and raise the heat so that the soup will start to boil.

5. Lower the heat to a simmer and allow it to cook for 15 minutes or so. Add in the chicken.

6. Optional: remove half of the mixture and pulse it for a few seconds using a stick blender. This is a great way to thicken the soup and promote flavor.

7. Put the soup back afterwards. However, if you don't have a stick blender, you can skip this step entirely.

8. Mix the olive oil with lemon juice and put it in the soup.

9. Place the fresh parsley and season the soup according to your taste.

Nutrition: Calories: 286 - **Carbohydrates:** 10.2g - **Protein:** 29g

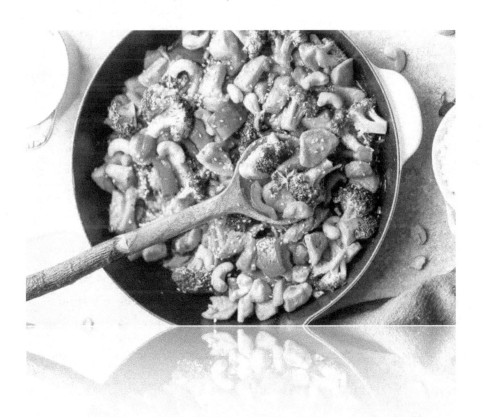

Keto Low Carb Vegetable

Preparation Time: 10 minutes

Cooking Time: 35 minutes

Servings: 12

Ingredients:

- 2 tbsp. of olive oil

- 1 tbsp. of Italian seasoning

- 2 cups of green beans (cut into 1-inch pieces)

- 8 cups of chicken broth

- 1 large onion (diced)

- 2 large bell peppers (diced)

- 4 cloves of garlic

- 1 medium head of cauliflower

- 2 14.5-oz cans of diced tomatoes

- Salt and pepper to taste

Kitchen Equipment:

- pot

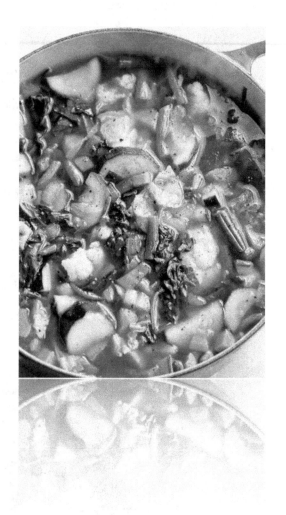

Directions:

1. Cook olive oil over medium heat using a pot. Put in the bell pepper and onions. Cook for 10 minutes or until the onions become browned. Put in the garlic and cook until fragrant.

2. Place the 8 cups of chicken broth. Add the green beans, cauliflower, broth, diced tomatoes, and Italian seasoning. Add salt and pepper to taste

3. Increase the heat and have the soup boiling before reducing it to a simmer and putting a lid on top.

4. The soup is ready when the green beans are already soft and ready for consumption. Enjoy!

Nutrition: Calories: 79 - **Fat:** 2g - **Protein:** 2g

Instant Pot Chili Verde

Preparation Time: 10 minutes

Cooking Time: 40 minutes

Servings: 4

Ingredients:

- 2 lbs. of boneless skinless chicken thighs
- 12 oz. of tomatillos (husked and quartered)
- 8 oz. of poblano peppers (stemmed, seeded, and chopped)
- 4 oz. of jalapeño peppers (stemmed, seeded, and chopped)
- 4 oz. of onions (chopped)
- 1/4 cup of water
- 1 1/2 tsp. of salt
- 2 tsp. of ground cumin
- 5 cloves of garlic
- ¼ oz. of chopped cilantro leaves (for finishing)
- 1 tbsp. of fresh lime juice (for finishing)

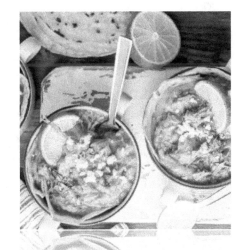

Kitchen Equipment:

- pressure cooker

Directions:

1. Put the poblanos, jalapenos, onions, and tomatillos in a pressure cooker.
2. Add the water and sprinkle the cumin, salt, and garlic on top.
3. Put the chicken inside and seal the lid.
4. Turn the pressure on high for 15 minutes.
5. Release the pressure and uncover the lid.
6. Put the chicken on a cutting board and cut it into small pieces. Set it aside.
7. Stir in cilantro and lime juice to the pressure cooker.
8. Choose the sauté mode on the pressure cooker.
9. Put the chicken back to the mixture and boil for the next 10 minutes to cause the chicken sauce to thicken. Stir it occasionally.
10. Serve and garnish with more cilantro if you want.

Nutrition:

Calories: 310 - **Total fat:** 15g - **Total carbohydrates:** 10g

Low-Carb Almond Coconut Sandie

Preparation Time: 15 minutes

Cooking Time: 12 minutes

Servings: 18

Ingredients:

- 1/3 tsp. of stevia powder
- 1 cup of coconut (unsweetened)
- 1 tsp. of Himalayan sea salt
- 1 cup of almond meal
- 1 tbsp. of vanilla extract
- 1/3 cup of melted coconut oil
- 2 tbsp. of water
- 1 egg white

Kitchen Equipment:

- oven
- parchment paper
- large bowl
- baking sheet
- wire rack

Directions:

1. Preheat the oven at 325 degrees F before you begin this dish. In addition to that, prepare a baking sheet by lining it with parchment paper.

2. Get a large bowl and put your Himalayan sea salt, unsweetened coconut, stevia powder, almond meal, vanilla extract, coconut oil, water, and egg white in it.

3. Stir this mixture properly. Set the bowl aside for 10 minutes. This is so that the unsweetened coconut will get considerably softer.

4. Mold the mixture into little balls. They should be small enough to fit on a tablespoon.

5. Place each ball on the prepared baking sheet. There should be some space between them.

6. Press down on the balls using a fork, slowly. As you don't want the edges to fall off.

7. Place the baking sheet in your oven and let the Sandie bake for about 15 minutes.

8. After letting the baking sheet cool for a minute, place it on a wire rack to get even cooler.

Nutrition:

Calories: 107 - **Protein:** 1.9g - **Fat:** 10.5g

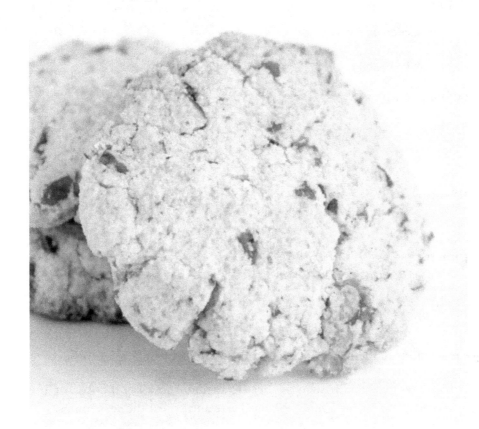

Pork Medallions with Cabbage

Preparation Time: 20 minutes

Cooking Time: 15 minutes

Servings: 2

Ingredients:

Ingredients

1ounce bacon, diced

2 pork medallions

2 garlic cloves, sliced

1 red onion, chopped

1 jalapeno pepper, deseeded and chopped

1 tablespoon apple cider vinegar

1/2 cup chicken bone broth

1/3-pound red cabbage, shredded

1 bay leaf

1 sprig rosemary

1 sprig thyme

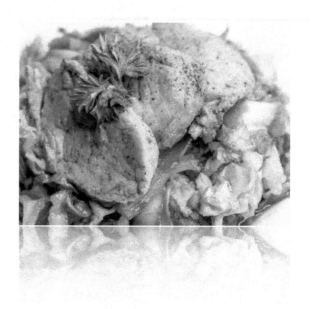

Kitchen Equipment:

frying pan

Directions:

Cook the pork medallions in the bacon grease until they are browned on both sides.

Add the remaining ingredients and reduce the heat to medium-low. Let it cook for 13 minutes more, gently stirring periodically to ensure even cooking. Taste and adjust the seasonings.

Nutrition:

Calories 528

Fat 31.8g

Protein 51.2g

Zingy Lemon Fish

Preparation Time: 50 minutes

Cooking Time: 40 minutes

Servings: 4

Ingredients:

14 ounces fresh Gurnard fish fillets

2 tablespoons lemon juice

6 tablespoons butter

½ cup fine almond flour

2 teaspoons dried chives

1 teaspoon garlic powder

2 teaspoons dried dill

2 teaspoons onion powder

Salt and pepper to taste

Kitchen Equipment:

large plate

large pan

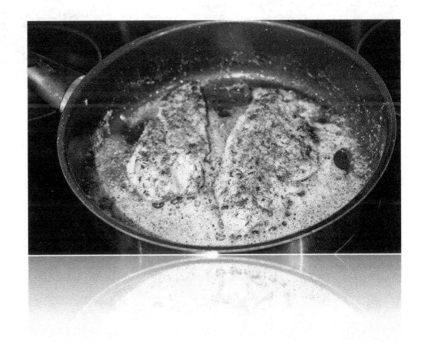

Directions:

Add almond flour, dried herbs, salt, and spices on a large plate and stir until well combined. Spread it all over the plate evenly.

Place a large pan over medium-high heat. Add half the butter and half the lemon juice. When butter just melts, place fillets on the pan and cook for 3 minutes. Move the fillets around the pan so that it absorbs the butter and lemon juice.

Add remaining half butter and lemon juice. When butter melts, flip sides and cook the other side for 3 minutes. Serve fillets with any butter remaining in the pan.

Nutrition: Calories 406 - **Fat** 30.3g - **Protein** 29g

Creamy Keto Fish Casserole

Preparation Time: 40 minutes
Cooking Time: 50 minutes
Servings: 4
Ingredients:

25 ounces of white fish (slice into bite-sized pieces)

15 ounces broccoli (small florets)

3 ounces butter + extra

6 scallions (finely chopped)

1 1/4 cups heavy whipping cream

2 tablespoons small capers

1 tablespoon dried parsley

1 tablespoon Dijon mustard

1/4 teaspoon black pepper (ground)

1 teaspoon salt

2 tablespoons olive oil

5 ounces leafy greens (finely chopped), for garnishing

Kitchen Equipment:

oven

saucepan

baking tray

Directions:

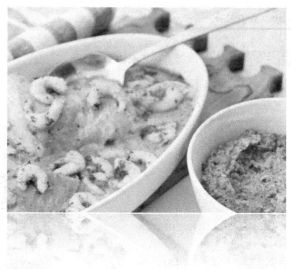

Preheat the oven to 400 degrees Fahrenheit. Cook the oil in a saucepan over medium-high heat.

Fry the broccoli florets in the hot oil for 5 minutes until tender and golden.

Transfer the fried florets to a small bowl and season it with salt and pepper. Toss the contents to ensure all the florets get an equal amount of seasoning.

Add the chopped scallions and capers to the same saucepan and fry for 2 minutes. Return the florets to the pan and mix well.

Grease a baking tray with a little amount of butter and spread the fried veggies (broccoli, scallions, and capers) in the baking tray.

Add the sliced fish to the tray and nestle it among the veggies.

Mix the heavy cream, mustard, and parsley in a small bowl and pour this mixture over the fish-veggie mixture. Top this with the remaining butter and spread gently over the contents using a spatula. Transfer to a plate and garnish with chopped greens. Serve warm and enjoy!

Nutrition: Calories 822 - Fat 69g - Protein 41g

Keto Fish Casserole with Mushrooms and French Mustard

Preparation Time: 40 minutes

Cooking Time: 50 minutes

Servings: 6

Ingredients:

25 ounces of white fish

15 ounces mushrooms (cut into wedges)

20 ounces cauliflower (cut into florets)

2 cups heavy whipping cream

3 ounces butter

2 tablespoons Dijon mustard

3 ounces olive oil

8 ounces cheese (shredded)

2 tablespoons fresh parsley

Salt & pepper, to taste

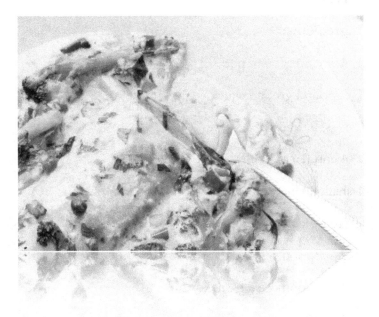

Kitchen Equipment:

oven

saucepan

Directions:

Prepare the oven to 350 degrees Fahrenheit Fry the mushroom for 5 minutes until tender and soft. Add the parsley, salt, and pepper to the mushrooms as you continue to mix well. Reduce the heat and add the mustard and heavy whipping cream to the mushroom.

Allow it simmer for 10 minutes until the sauce thickens and reduces a bit. Season the fish slices with pepper and salt. Set aside.

Sprinkle 3/4th of the cheese over the fish slices and spread the creamy mushroom over the top. Now again, top it with the remaining cheese.

Boil the cauliflower florets in lightly salted water for 5 minutes and strain the water. Place the strained florets in a bowl and add the olive oil. Mash thoroughly with a fork until you get a coarse texture—season with salt and pepper. Mix well.

Nutrition: Calories 828 - **Fat** 71g - **Protein** 39g

Festive Meatloaf

Preparation Time: 1 hour

Cooking Time: 50 minutes

Servings: 2

Ingredients:

1/4-pound ground pork

1/2-pound ground chuck

2 eggs, beaten

1/4 cup flaxseed meal

1 shallot, chopped

2 garlic cloves, minced

1/2 teaspoon smoked paprika

1/4 teaspoon dried basil

1/4 teaspoon ground cumin

Kosher salt, to taste

1/2 cup tomato puree

1 teaspoon mustard

1 teaspoon liquid monk fruit

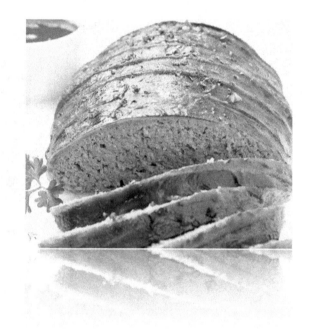

Kitchen Equipment:

2 mixing bowl

loaf pan

oven

Directions:

In a bowl, mix thoroughly the ground meat, eggs, flaxseed meal, shallot, garlic, and spices.

In another bowl, mix the tomato puree with the mustard and liquid monk fruit, whisk to combine well.

Press the mixture into the loaf pan—Bake in the preheated oven at 360 degrees F for 30 minutes.

Nutrition: Calories 517 - **Fat** 32.3g - **Protein** 48.5g

Rich Winter Beef Stew

Preparation Time: 45 minutes

Cooking Time: 50 minutes

Servings: 2

Ingredients:

1-ounce bacon, diced

3/4-pound well-marbled beef chuck, boneless and cut into 1-1/2-inch pieces

1 red bell pepper, chopped

1 green bell pepper, chopped

2 garlic cloves, minced

1/2 cup leeks, chopped

1 parsnip, chopped

Sea salt, to taste

1/4 teaspoon mixed peppercorns, freshly cracked

2 cups of chicken bone broth

1 tomato, pureed

2 cups kale, torn into pieces

1 tablespoon fresh cilantro, roughly chopped

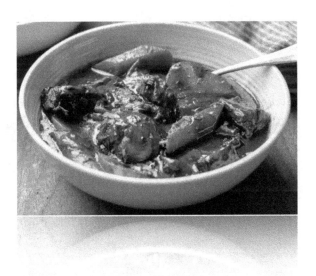

Kitchen Equipment:

Dutch pot

Directions:

Heat a Dutch pot over medium-high flame. Now, cook the bacon until it is well browned and crisp; reserve. Then, cook the beef pieces for 3 to 5 minutes or until just browned on all sides; reserve. After that, sauté the peppers, garlic, leeks, and parsnip in the pan drippings until they are just tender and aromatic. Add the salt, peppercorns, chicken bone broth, tomato, and reserved beef to the pot. Bring to a boil. Stir in the kale leaves and continue simmering until the leaves have wilted or 3 to 4 minutes more.

Ladle into individual bowls and serve garnished with fresh cilantro and the reserved bacon.

Nutrition: - Calories 359 **- Fat** 17.8g **- Fiber** 1g

Mini Meatloaves with Spinach

Preparation Time: 35 minutes

Cooking Time: 40 minutes

Servings: 2

Ingredients:

1/2-pound lean ground beef

2 tablespoons tomato paste

1 teaspoon Dijon mustard

1 egg, beaten

1/2 teaspoon ginger garlic paste

1/2 cup shallots, finely chopped

1 tablespoon canola oil

1/2 teaspoon coconut amino

1/4 cup almond meal

1 bunch spinach, chopped

1 teaspoon dried parsley flakes

1/2 teaspoon dried basil

1/2 teaspoon dried rosemary

1/2 teaspoon dried sage

1/4 teaspoon cayenne pepper

Kosher salt and ground black pepper

2 tablespoons sour cream

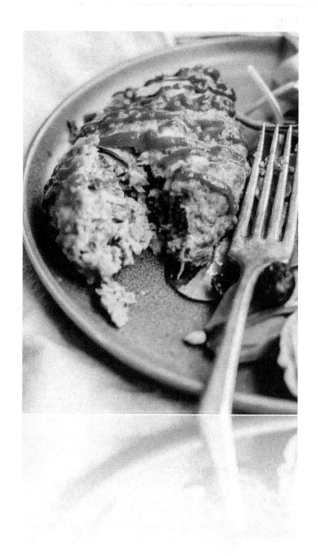

Kitchen Equipment:

muffin tin

oven

Directions:

Place the meat mixture into a lightly greased muffin tin. Bake the mini meatloaves in the preheated oven at 360 degrees F for 20 to 28 minutes.

Serve with sour cream and enjoy!

Nutrition: Calories 434 - **Fat** 29.4g - **Protein** 37.1g

Keto Thai Fish with Curry and Coconut

Preparation Time: 50 minutes

Cooking Time: 40 minutes

Servings: 4

Ingredients:

25 ounces salmon (slice into bite-sized pieces)

15 ounces cauliflower (bite-sized florets)

14 ounces coconut cream

1-ounce olive oil

4 tablespoons butter

Salt and pepper, to taste

Kitchen Equipment:

oven

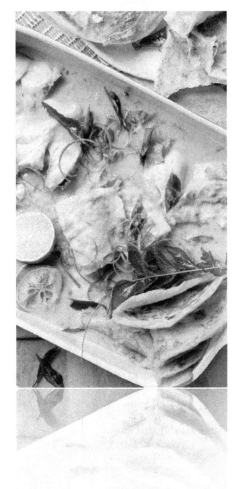

Directions:

Prepare the oven to 400 degrees Fahrenheit Sprinkle salt and pepper over the salmon generously. Toss it once, if possible. Place the butter generously over all the salmon pieces and set aside.

Pour this cream mixture over the fish in the baking tray. Meanwhile, boil the cauliflower florets in salted water for 5 minutes, strain and mash the florets coarsely. Set aside. Transfer the creamy fish to a plate and serve with mashed cauliflower. Enjoy!

Nutrition:

Calories 880

Fat 75g

Protein 42g

Keto Salmon Tandoori with Cucumber Sauce

Preparation Time: 10 minutes

Cooking Time: 50 minutes

Servings: 4

Ingredients

25 ounces salmon (bite-sized pieces)

2 tablespoons coconut oil

1 tablespoon tandoori seasoning

For the cucumber sauce

1/2 shredded cucumber (squeeze out the water completely)

Juice of 1/2 lime

2 minced garlic cloves

1 1/4 cups sour cream or mayonnaise

1/2 teaspoon salt (optional)

For the crispy salad

3 1/2 ounces lettuce (torn)

3 scallions (finely chopped)

2 avocados (cubed)

1 yellow bell pepper (diced)

Juice of 1 lime

Kitchen Equipment:

oven

2 small bowl

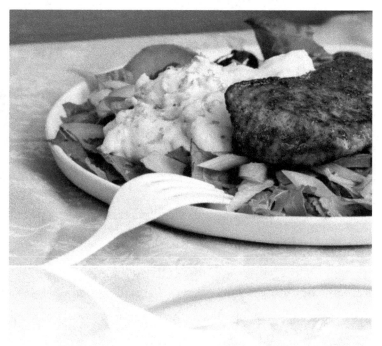

Directions:

Preheat the oven to 350 degrees Fahrenheit Mix the tandoori seasoning with oil in a small bowl and coat the salmon pieces with this mixture. Bake for 20 minutes until soft and the salmon flakes with a fork

Take another bowl and place the shredded cucumber in it. Add the mayonnaise, minced garlic, and salt (if the mayonnaise doesn't have salt) to the shredded cucumber.

Mix the lettuce, scallions, avocados, and bell pepper in another bowl. Drizzle the contents with the lime juice.

Transfer the veggie salad to a plate and place the baked salmon over it. Top the veggies and salmon with cucumber sauce. Serve immediately and enjoy!

Nutrition: Calories 847 - **Fat** 73g - **Protein** 35g

Mocha Crunch Oatmeal

Preparation Time: 15 minutes

Cooking Time: 5 minutes

Servings: 4

Ingredients:

1 cup of steel-cut oats

1 1/2 cup of cocoa powder

1 cup of cinnamon

1/4 teaspoon salt

2 cups of sugar

1/4 cup of agave nectar roasted mixed nuts

1/4 cup of bittersweet chocolate chips Milk or cream to serve.

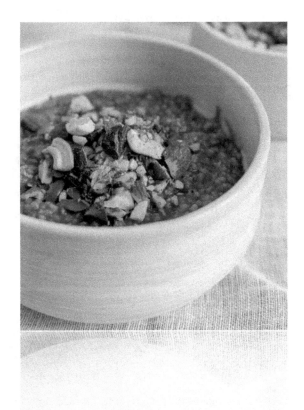

Kitchen Equipment:

saucepan

Directions:

Bring water to a boil. Stir in oats, cocoa powder, espresso, and salt. Bring to a boil again and raising heat to medium-low. Simmer uncovered for 20 to 30 minutes, frequently stirring until the oats hit the tenderness you need. Remove from heat and whisk in sugar or agave nectar.

While the oatmeal cooks, the mixed nuts and chocolate chips roughly chop. Place them in a small bowl to eat.

Serve with hot milk or cream on the side when the oatmeal is full, and sprinkle liberally with a coating of nut and chocolate.

Nutrition: calories 118 - **fat** 12g - **protein** 26g

Keto Sausage Breakfast Sandwich

Preparation Time: 5 minutes

Cooking Time: 15 minutes

Servings: 3

Ingredients:

6 large eggs

2 tbsp. heavy cream

Pinch red pepper flakes

Kosher salt

Freshly ground black pepper

1 tbsp. butter

3 slices cheddar

6 frozen sausage patties, heated according to package instructions

Avocado, sliced

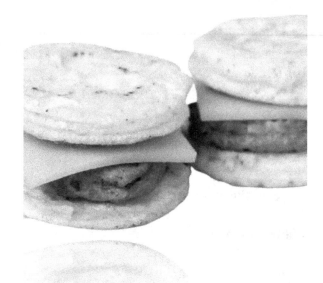

Kitchen Equipment:

small bowl

nonstick container

Directions:

Beat the eggs, heavy cream, and red pepper flakes together in a small bowl.

Heat butter in a non-stick container over medium flame. Pour 1/3 of the eggs into your skillet. Place a cheese slice in the center and allow it to sit for about 1 minute. Fold the egg sides in the middle, covering the cheese. Remove from saucepan and repeat with eggs left over.

Serve the eggs with avocado in between two sausage patties.

Nutrition: Calories 113 - **Fats** 10g - **Protein** 27g

Cabbage Hash Browns

Preparation Time: 10 minutes

Cooking Time: 25 minutes

Servings: 2

Ingredients:

2 large eggs

1/2 tsp. garlic powder

1/2 tsp. kosher salt

Freshly ground black pepper

2 c. shredded cabbage

1/4 small yellow onion, thinly sliced

1 tbsp. vegetable oil

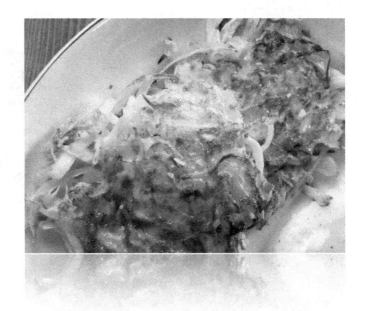

Kitchen Equipment:

large bowl

blender

large skillet

spatula

Directions:

Whisk shells, eggs, garlic powder, and salt together in a large bowl. Season with black potatoes. Add the chicken and onion to the mixture of the eggs and blend together.

Cook oil in a large skillet over medium to high heat. In the pan, divide the mixture into four patties and press to flatten with the spatula. Cook side, until golden and tender.

Nutrition: Calories 109 - **Fats** 9g - **Protein** 21g

Keto Breakfast Cups

Preparation Time: 15 minutes

Cooking Time: 40 minutes

Servings: 12

Ingredients:

2 lb. ground pork

1 tbsp. freshly chopped thyme

2 cloves garlic, minced

1/2 tsp. paprika

1/2 tsp. ground cumin

1 tsp. kosher salt

Freshly ground black pepper

2 1/2 c. chopped fresh spinach

1 c. shredded white cheddar

12 eggs

1 tbsp. freshly chopped chives

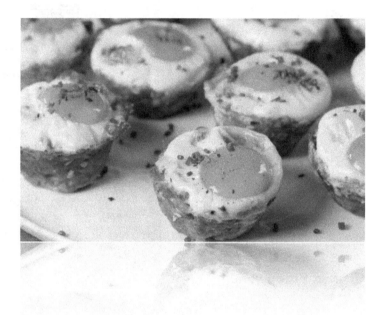

Kitchen Equipment:

oven

muffin tin

Directions:

Oven preheats to 400 ° c. combine the soiled pork, thyme, garlic, paprika, cumin, and salt in a large bowl. Season with peppers.

Attach a small handful of pork to each tin of muffin well then press the sides to make a cup. Spinach and cheese should be evenly divided between cups. Season with salt and pepper and crack an egg on top of each cup.

Bake for about 25 minutes, until eggs are set, and sausage is cooked through. Garnish and serve with chives.

Nutrition: Calories 117 - **Fat** 14g - **Protein** 30g

Egg Salad

Preparation Time: 15 minutes

Cooking Time: 20 minutes

Servings: 6

Ingredients:

3 tbsp. mayonnaise

3 tbsp. Greek yogurt

2 tbsp. red wine vinegar

Kosher salt

Freshly ground black pepper

8 hard-boiled eggs, cut into eight pieces

8 strips bacon, cooked and crumbled

1 avocado, thinly sliced

1/2 c. crumbled blue cheese

1/2 c. cherry tomatoes

2 tbsp. freshly chopped chives

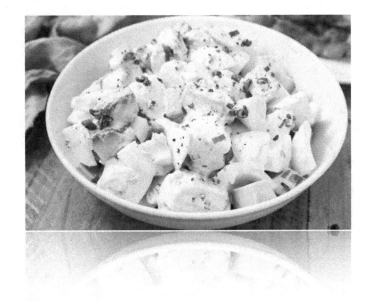

Kitchen Equipment:

small bowl

large bowl

Directions:

Stir mayonnaise, cream, and the red wine vinegar in a small bowl. Season with pepper and salt.

Kindly combine the eggs, bacon, avocado, blue cheese, and cherry tomatoes in a large serving bowl. Gradually fold in the mayonnaise dressing until the ingredients are coated slightly, then season with salt and pepper. Garnish with the chives and extra toppings.

Nutrition: Calories 110 - **Fats** 10g - **Protein** 26g

Taco Stuffed Avocados

Preparation Time: 10 minutes

Cooking Time: 25 minutes

Servings: 8

Ingredients:

4ripe avocados

Juice of 1 lime

1 tbsp. extra-virgin olive oil

1medium onion, chopped

1 lb. ground beef

1 packet taco seasoning

Kosher salt

Freshly ground black pepper

2/3 c. shredded Mexican cheese

1/2 c. shredded lettuce

1/2 c. quartered grape tomatoes

Sour cream, for topping

Kitchen Equipment:

medium skillet

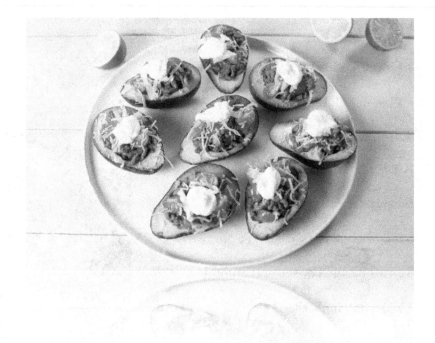

Directions:

Half and the pit avocados. Scoop a bit of avocado out using a spoon, creating a bigger well. Dice have removed avocado and set aside for later use. Squeeze lime juice (to avoid browning!) overall avocados.

Heat oil in a medium-sized skillet over medium heat. Add onion, and cook for about 5 minutes, until tender. Attach ground beef and taco seasoning, with a wooden spoon breaking up the meat. Season well and cook for about 6 minutes until the beef is no longer pink. Take off heat and drain fat.

Fill every half of the avocado with beef, then top with reserved avocado, cheese, lettuce, tomato, and a sour dollop cream.

Nutrition: Calories 107 - **Fat** 11g - **Protein** 30g

Buffalo Shrimp Lettuce Wraps

Preparation Time: 15 minutes

Cooking Time: 20 minutes

Servings: 4

Ingredients:

1/4 tbsp. butter

2 garlic cloves, minced

1/4 c. hot sauce, such as Frank's

1 tbsp. extra-virgin olive oil

1 lb. shrimp, peeled and deveined, tails removed

Kosher salt

Freshly ground black pepper

1 head romaine leaf separated, for serving

1/4 red onion, finely chopped

1 rib celery, sliced thin

1/2 c. blue cheese, crumbled

Kitchen Equipment:

saucepan

large skillet

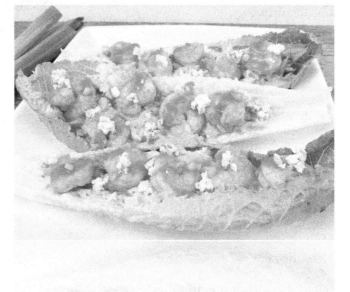

Directions:

Make buffalo sauce: melt butter over medium heat in a small saucepan. When completely melted, add the garlic and cook for 1 minute until it is fragrant. Attach hot sauce to combine, and stir. Switch heat to low while the shrimp are cooking.

Make shrimp: heat oil in a large skillet over medium heat. Add shrimp, and add salt and pepper to season. Cook, flipping halfway, till both sides are pink and opaque, around 2 minutes per side turn off the heat and apply the sauce to the buffalo, tossing to coat.

Assemble wraps: add a small scoop of shrimp to a roman leaf center, then top with red onion, celery, and blue cheese.

Nutrition: Calories 108 - **Fats** 8g - **Protein** 26g

Broccoli Bacon Salad

Preparation Time: 15 minutes

Cooking Time: 15 minutes

Servings: 6

Ingredients:

For the salad:

kosher salt 3

heads broccoli, cut into bite-size pieces

Two carrots, shredded

1/2 red onion, thinly sliced

1/2 c. dried cranberries

1/2 c. sliced almonds

6 slices bacon, cooked and crumbled

For the dressing:

1/2 c. mayonnaise

3 tbsp. apple cider vinegar

kosher salt

Freshly ground black pepper

Kitchen Equipment:

medium sauce pan

large bowl

colander

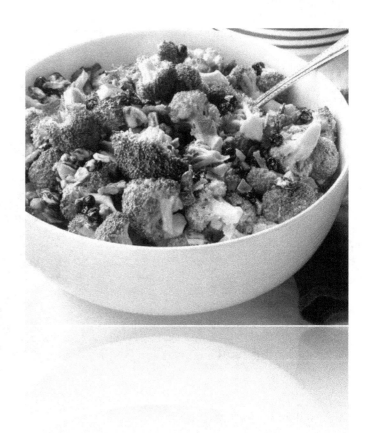

Directions:

Bring 4 cups of salted water up to a boil in a medium saucepan. Prepare a large bowl of ice water while waiting for the water to boil.

Add broccoli florets to the heated water, and cook for 1 to 2 minutes until tender. Remove with a slotted spoon and put the ice water in the prepared cup. Drain flourishes within a colander when cold.

Combine broccoli, red onion, carrots, cranberries, nuts, and bacon in a large bowl. Whisk vinegar and mayonnaise together in a medium bowl and season with salt and pepper. Pour the broccoli mixture over the dressing and stir to combine.

Nutrition: Calories 116 **- Fats** 12g **- Protein** 37g

Keto Salad

Preparation Time: 15 minutes

Cooking Time: 15 minutes

Servings: 4

Ingredients:

3 tbsp. mayonnaise

2 tsp. lemon juice

1 tbsp. finely chopped chives

Freshly ground black pepper

Kosher salt

6 hard-boiled eggs, peeled and chopped

1 avocado, cubed

Lettuce, for serving

Cooked bacon, for serving

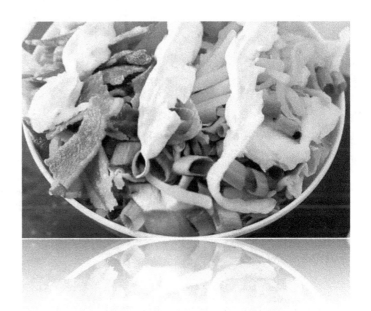

Kitchen Equipment:

medium bowl

Directions:

Whisk the mayonnaise, lemon juice, and chives together in a medium bowl. Season with pepper and salt. Add eggs and avocado to mix and throw gently. Serve with Bacon and Lettuce.

Nutrition:

Calories 114 - **Fat** 9g - **Protein** 30g

Keto Bacon Sushi

Preparation Time: 10 minutes

Cooking Time: 30 minutes

Servings: 12

Ingredients:

6 slices bacon halved

2 Persian cucumbers, thinly sliced

2 medium carrots, thinly sliced

1 avocado, sliced

4 oz. cream cheese softened

Sesame seeds, for garnish

Kitchen Equipment:

oven

aluminum foil

baking sheet

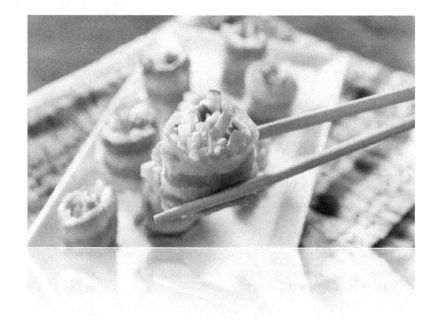

Directions:

Preheat oven to around 400o. Strip an aluminum foil baking sheet and fit it with a refrigerating rack. Lay the bacon halves in an even layer and bake for 11 to 13 minutes, until slightly crisp yet pliable. In the meantime, the cucumbers, carrots, and avocado are sliced into parts around the bacon width.

Place one even layer of cream cheese on each slice when the bacon is cool enough to touch. Equally, divide vegetables between the bacon and put them on one end. Roll up tightly on vegetables.

Garnish, and serve with sesame seeds

Nutrition: Calories 109 - **Fat** 10g - **Protein** 27g

Loaded Cauliflower Salad

Preparation Time: 10 minutes

Cooking Time: 30 minutes

Servings: 6

Ingredients:

1 large head cauliflower, cut into florets

6 slices bacon

1/2 c. sour cream

1/4 c. mayonnaise

1 tbsp. lemon juice

1/2 tsp. garlic powder

Kosher salt

Freshly ground black pepper

1 1/2 c. shredded cheddar

1/4 c. finely chopped chives

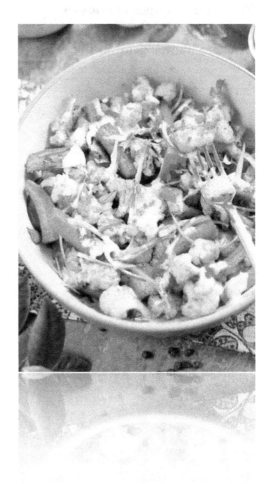

Kitchen Equipment:

large skillet

Directions:

Bring around ¼ cup of water into a large skillet to boil. Add cauliflower, cover pan and steam for about 4 minutes, until tender. Drain and allow to cool while preparing other ingredients.

Start cooking the pork in a pan over medium heat, around 3 minutes per side, until crispy. Switch to a towel-lined sheet of paper for drain, then cut.

Whisk the sour cream, mayonnaise, lemon juice, and garlic powder together in a big bowl. Remove cauliflower and gently toss. Add salt and pepper, then fold into bacon, cheddar, and chives. Serve warm, or at ambient temperature.

Nutrition: Calories 440 - **Fat** 135g - **Protein** 26g

Caprese Zoodles

Preparation Time: 10 minutes

Cooking Time: 25 minutes

Servings: 4

Ingredients:

4 large zucchinis

2 tbsp. extra-virgin olive oil

kosher salt

Freshly ground black pepper

2 c. cherry tomatoes halved

1 c. mozzarella balls, quartered if large

1/4 c. fresh basil leaves

2 tbsp. balsamic vinegar

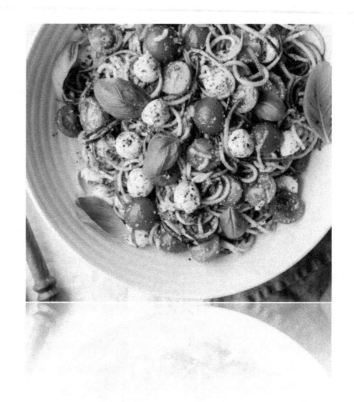

Kitchen Equipment:

spiralizer

large bowl

Directions:

Creating zoodles out of zucchini using a spiralizer. In a large bowl, add the zoodles, mix with the olive oil and season with the salt and pepper. Let them marinate for 15 minutes.

In zoodles, add the tomatoes, mozzarella, and basil and toss until combined. Drizzle, and drink with balsamic.

Nutrition: - **Calories** 116 - **Fat** 115g - **Protein** 31g

Chicken Spinach Curry

Preparation Time: 10 minutes

Cooking Time: 17 minutes

Servings: 4

Ingredients:

2 tomatoes, chopped

4 ounces spinach, chopped

1/3-pound curry paste

1 1/2 cups yogurt

4 pounds chicken, cubed

1 tablespoon olive oil

1 onion, cut to make slices

1 tablespoon chopped coriander

Kitchen Equipment:

mixing bowl

instant pot

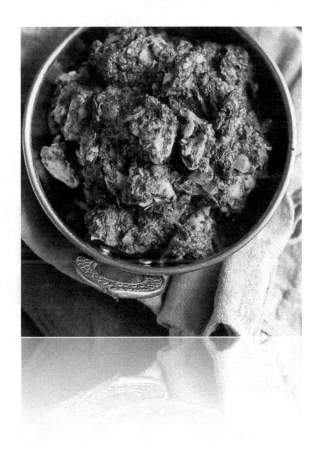

Directions:

Combine the chicken, curry paste, and yogurt in a mixing bowl. Wrap and soak in the fridge for 30 minutes. Situate the Instant Pot over a dry surface in your kitchen. Open and turn it on.

Click "SAUTE" cooking function; pour the oil in it and allow it to heat. In the pot, stir in the onions; cook (while stirring) until turns translucent and softened. Mix the tomatoes and cook for another minute.

Pour the chicken mixture, mix in the spinach and coriander; gently stir to mix well. Close the lid. Select "MANUAL" cooking function; timer to 15 minutes with default "HIGH" pressure mode.

Let the pressure to build to cook the ingredients. After cooking time is over click "CANCEL". Set "QPR" cooking function. This setting is for quick release of inside pressure.

Gradually open the lid, put the cooked dish in the serving plates.

Nutrition:

Calories 384 - **Fat** 18g - **Protein** 12g

Super Herbed Fish

Preparation Time: 10 minutes

Cooking Time: 6 minutes

Servings: 1

Ingredients:

1 tablespoon chopped basil

2 teaspoons lime zest

1 tablespoon lime juice

1 tablespoon olive oil

1 4-ounce fish fillet

1 rosemary sprig

1 thyme sprig

1 teaspoon Dijon mustard

¼ teaspoon garlic powder

Pinch of salt

Pinch of pepper

1 ½ cups water

Kitchen Equipment:

parchment paper

mixing bowl

aluminum foil

instant pot

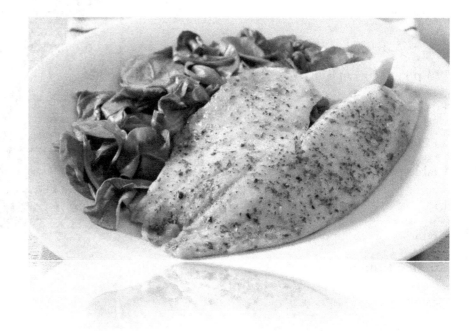

Directions:

Season the fish with salt and paper. Wrap a piece of parchment paper and sprinkle with zest. Whisk together the oil, juice, and mustard in a mixing bowl and brush over. Top with the herbs. Wrap the fish with the parchment paper. Wrap the wrapped fish in an aluminum foil. Get the Instant Pot in platform in your kitchen. Open and switch it on. In the pot, pour water. Arrange a trivet or steamer basket inside that came with Instant Pot. Now place/arrange the foil over the trivet/basket.

Close the lid.

Press "MANUAL" cooking function; timer to 5 minutes with default "HIGH" pressure mode. Let the pressure to build to cook the ingredients.

After cooking time is over select "CANCEL". Adjust to "QPR" cooking function. For fast release of inside pressure. Lightly open the lid, take out the cooked recipe in serving bowls.

Nutrition: Calories 246 - Fat 9g - Carbohydrates 1g

Turkey Avocado Chili

Preparation Time: 10 minutes

Cooking Time: 50 minutes

Servings: 4

Ingredients:

2 ½ pounds lean (finely ground) turkey

2 cups diced tomatoes

2-ounce tomato paste, sugar-free

1 tablespoon olive oil

½ chopped large yellow onion

8 minced garlic cloves

1 (4-ounce) can green chilies with liquid

2 tablespoons Worcestershire sauce

1 tablespoon dried oregano

¼ cup red chili powder

2 tablespoons (finely ground) cumin

Salt and freshly (finely ground) black pepper, as per taste preference

1 pitted and sliced avocado, peeled

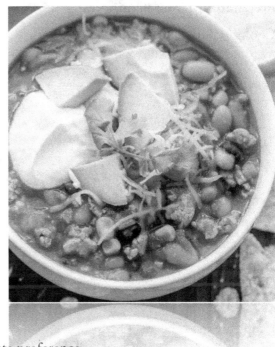

Kitchen Equipment:

Instant pot

Directions:

Place the Instant Pot over a dry podium in your kitchen. Switch it on.

Select "SAUTE" cooking function; fill the oil in it and allow it to heat.

In the pot, mix the onions; cook (while stirring) until turns translucent and softened for around 4-5 minutes.

Add the garlic and cook for about 1 minute.

Add the turkey and cook for about 8-9 minutes. Stir in remaining ingredients except for the avocado.

Close the lid.

Choose "MEAT/STEW" cooking function; timer to 35 minutes with default "HIGH" pressure mode.

Allow the pressure to build to cook the ingredients.

After cooking time is over click "CANCEL". Set to "NPR" cooking function for the natural release, and it takes around 10 minutes to release pressure slowly.

Gradually open the lid, pull out the cooked dish and place in serving plates, top with the avocado slices, and enjoy the Keto recipe.

Nutrition: Calories 346 **- Fat** 19g **- Fiber** 5g

Cheesy Tomato Shrimp

Preparation Time: 10 minutes

Cooking Time: 15 minutes

Servings: 4

Ingredients:

2 tablespoons olive oil

½ cup veggie broth

¼ cup chopped cilantro

2 tablespoons lime juice

1 ½ pounds shrimp, peeled and deveined

1 ½ pounds tomatoes, chopped

1 jalapeno, diced

1 onion, diced

1 cup shredded cheddar cheese

1 teaspoon minced garlic

Kitchen Equipment:

Instant pot

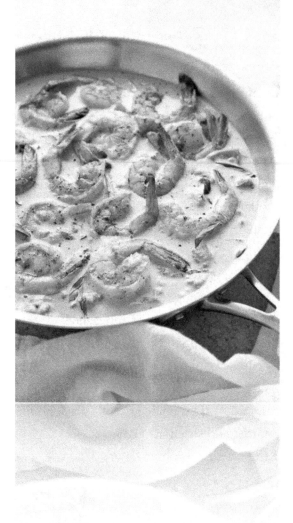

Directions:

Put the Instant Pot in a surface in your kitchen. Open its top lid and turn it on. Set "SAUTE" cooking function; put the oil in it and allow it to heat. In the pot, place the onions; cook (while stirring) until turns translucent and softened for around 2-3 minutes.

Add garlic and sauté for 30-60 seconds. Stir in the broth, cilantro, and tomatoes and secure the lid

Find and press "MANUAL" cooking function; timer to 9 minutes with default "HIGH" pressure mode. Let the pressure cook the ingredients.

After cooking time is over press "CANCEL". set "NPR" cooking function for the release, for around 10 minutes to release pressure slowly.

Add the shrimps. Close the top lid. Find and press "MANUAL" cooking function; timer to 2 minutes with default "HIGH" pressure mode.

Let the pressure to build to cook the ingredients. After cooking time is over select "CANCEL". Then press "NPR" cooking function for the release of inside pressure, and for around 10 minutes to release pressure slowly.

Slowly transfer the cooked meals into serving bowls, top with the cheddar, and enjoy the Keto recipe.

Nutrition: Calories 268 **- Fat** 16g **- Carbohydrates** 7g

Cajun Rosemary Chicken

Preparation Time: 10 minutes

Cooking Time: 30 minutes

Servings: 4

Ingredients:

2 teaspoons Cajun seasoning

1 lemon, halved

1 yellow onion, make quarters

1 teaspoon garlic salt

1 medium chicken

2 rosemary sprigs

1 tablespoon coconut oil

1/4 teaspoon pepper

1 1/2 cups chicken broth

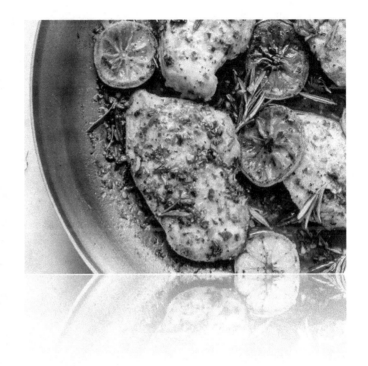

Kitchen Equipment:

Instant pot

Directions:

Season the chicken and Cajun seasoning. Stuff the lemon, onion, and rosemary in the chicken's cavity. Get the Instant Pot then open its top lid and turn it on.

Press "SAUTE" cooking function; place the oil in it and allow it to heat. Put the meat; cook (while stirring) until turns evenly brown from all sides. Add the broth; gently stir to mix well.

Close the lid then click "MANUAL" cooking function; timer to 25 minutes with default "HIGH" pressure mode.

Let the pressure to build to cook the ingredients. After cooking time is over press "CANCEL". Then "NPR" cooking function for the natural release of inside pressure, and for around 10 minutes to release pressure slowly.

Gradually open the lid, place dish in serving plates or serving bowls, and enjoy the Keto recipe.

Nutrition: Calories 236 - **Fat** 26g - **Fiber** 5g

Sriracha Tuna Kabobs

Preparation Time: 4 minutes

Cooking Time: 9 minutes

Servings: 4

Ingredients

4 tablespoon Huy Fong chili garlic sauce

1 tablespoon sesame oil infused with garlic

1 tablespoon ginger, fresh, grated

1 tablespoon garlic, minced

1 red onion, cut into quarters

2 cups bell peppers, red, green, yellow

1 can whole water chestnuts

½ pound fresh mushrooms halved

32 oz. boneless tuna, chunks or steaks

1 Splenda packet

2 zucchinis, sliced

1 inch thick, keep skins on

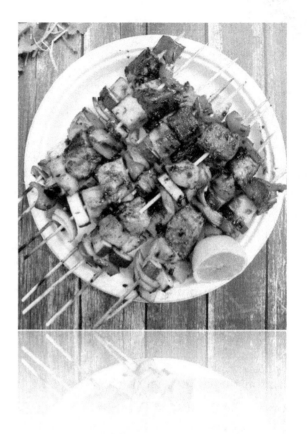

Kitchen Equipment:

skewers

blender

griller

Directions:

Layer the tuna and the vegetable pieces evenly onto 8 skewers. Combine the spices and the oil and chili sauce, add the Splenda Quickly blend, either in a blender or by Quickly whipping.

Brush onto the kabob pieces, make sure every piece is coated Grill 4 minutes on each district, check to ensure the tuna is cooked to taste. Serving size is two skewers.

Mix the marinade ingredients and store in a covered container in the fridge. Place all the vegetables in one container in the fridge. Place the tuna in a separate zip-lock bag.

Nutrition: Calories 467 **- Protein** 56g **- Fiber** 3.5g

Chicken Casserole

Preparation Time: 19 minutes

Cooking Time: 29 minutes

Servings: 4

Ingredients

6 Tortilla Factory low-carb whole wheat tortillas, torn into small pieces

1 ½ cups hand-shredded cheese, Mexican

1 beaten egg

1 cup milk

2 cups cooked chicken, shredded

1 can Ro-tel

½ cup salsa Verde

Kitchen Equipment:

8x8 glass baking dish

oven

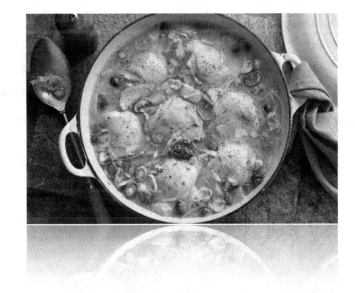

Directions:

Brush an 8 x 8 glass baking dish with oil. Heat oven to 375 degrees Combine everything, but reserve ½ cup8 x 8 glass baking tray with margarine. Heat oven to 375 degrees Combine everything, but reserve ½ cup of the cheese Bake it for 29 minutes

Take it out of the furnace and add ½ cup cheese Broil for about 2 minutes to melt the cheese Let the casserole cool. Slice into 6 slices and place in freezer containers, (1 cup with a lid) Fix. Microwave for 2 minutes to serve. Top with sour cream, if desired.

Nutrition: 265 **Calories** - 20g **Protein** - 10g **Fiber**

Steak with Spice Salad

Preparation Time: 4 minutes

Cooking Time: 4 minutes

Servings: 2

Ingredients

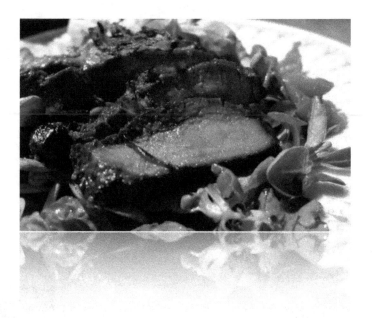

2 tablespoon sriracha sauce

1 tablespoon garlic, minced

1 tablespoon ginger, fresh, grated

1 bell pepper, yellow, cut into thin strips

1 bell pepper, red, cut into thin strips

1 tablespoon sesame oil, garlic

1 Splenda packet

½ tablespoon curry powder

½ tablespoon rice wine vinegar

8 oz. of beef sirloin, cut into strips

2 cups baby spinach, stemmed

½ head butter lettuce, torn or chopped into bite-sized pieces

Kitchen Equipment:

2 bowls

Directions:

Place the garlic, sriracha sauce, 1 tablespoon sesame oil, rice wine vinegar, and Splenda into a basin and combine nicely. Pour half of this mix into a zip-lock bag. Add the steak to marinade while you are preparing the salad. Assemble the brightly colored salad by layering in two bowls.

You must put in the spinach into the bottom of the bowl. Place the butter lettuce next. Mix the two peppers and place on top.

Remove the steak from the marinade and discard the liquid and bag.

Heat the sesame oil and rapidly stir fry the steak until desired doneness, it should have about 3 minutes. Situate the steak on top of the salad.

Drizzle with the remaining dressing (another field of marinade mix). Sprinkle sriracha sauce across the salad.

Combine the salad ingredients and stand in a zip-lock bag in the fridge. Mix the marinade and halve into 2 zip-lock bags. Place the sriracha sauce into a small sealed container. Slice the steak and freeze in a zip-lock bag with the marinade. To make, mix the ingredients like the initial Directions:. Stir fry the marinated beef for 4 minutes to take into consideration the beef is frozen.

Nutrition: Calories 350 - **Total Fat** 23g - **Protein** 28g

Chicken Chow Mein Stir Fry

Preparation Time: 9 minutes

Cooking Time: 14 minutes

Servings: 4

Ingredients

1/2 cup sliced onion

2 tablespoon Oil, sesame garlic flavored

4 cups shredded Bok-Choy

1 cup Sugar Snap Peas

1 cup fresh bean sprouts

3 stalks Celery, chopped

1 1/2 tablespoon minced Garlic

1 packet Splenda

1 cup Broth, chicken

2 tablespoon Soy Sauce

1 tablespoon ginger, freshly minced

1 tablespoon cornstarch

4 boneless Chicken Breasts, cooked/sliced thinly

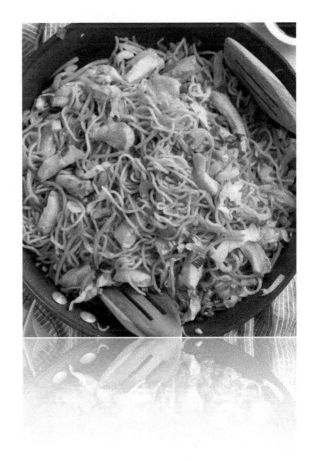

Kitchen Equipment:

skillet

Directions:

Place the bok-choy, peas, celery in a skillet with 1 T garlic oil. Stir fry until bok-choy is softened to liking. Add remaining ingredients except for the cornstarch.

If too thin, stir cornstarch into ½ cup lukewarm water when smooth flow into skillet. Bring cornstarch and chow Mein to a one-minute boil. Turn off the heat source. Stir sauce then wait for 4 minutes to serve, after the chow Mein has thickened.

Freeze in covered containers. Heat for 2 minutes in the microwave before serving.

Nutrition: Calories 368 - Total Fat 18g - Protein42g

Salmon with Bok-Choy

Preparation Time: 9 minutes

Cooking Time: 9 minutes

Servings: 4

Ingredients

1 cup red peppers, roasted, drained

2 cups chopped bok-choy

1 tablespoon salted butter

5 oz. salmon steak

1 lemon, sliced very thinly

1/8 tablespoon black pepper

1 tablespoon olive oil

2 tablespoon sriracha sauce

Kitchen Equipment:

skillet

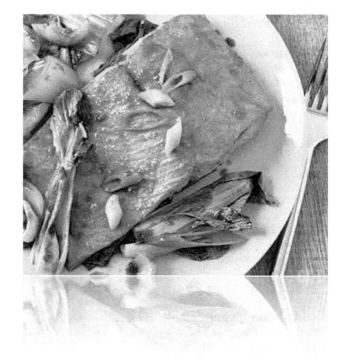

Directions:

Place oil in a skillet Place all but 4 slices of lemon in the skillet. Place the bok choy with the black pepper.

Stir fry the bok-choy with the lemons. Remove and place on four plates. Place the butter in the skillet and stir fry the salmon, turning once.

Place the salmon on the bed of bok-choy. Split the red peppers and encircle the salmon. Transfer a slice of lemon on top of the salmon.

Drizzle with sriracha sauce. Freeze the cooked salmon in individual zip-lock bags. Place the bok-choy, with the remaining ingredients into one-cup containers. Microwave the salmon for one minute and the frozen bok choy for two. Assemble to serve.

Nutrition: Calories 410 - **Total Fat** 30g - **Protein** 30g

Tortilla Breakfast Casserole

Preparation Time: 10 minutes

Cooking Time: 30 minutes

Servings: 12

Ingredients

1 Pound Bacon, Cooked and Crumbled

1 Pound Pork Sausage. Cooked and Crumbled

1 Pound Package Diced Ham

10 8-inch Tortillas, Cut in half 8 Large Eggs

1 1/2 Cups Milk

1/2 Teaspoon Salt

1/2 Teaspoon Pepper

1/2 Teaspoon Garlic Powder

1/2 teaspoon Hot Sauce

2 Cups Shredded Cheddar Cheese

1 Cup Mozzarella or Monterrey Jack Cheese

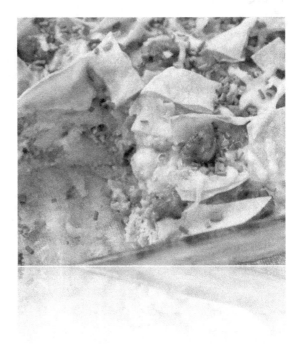

Kitchen Equipment:

9x13 baking dish

pan

large bowl

oven

Directions:

Grease 9x13-inch baking dish with 2 teaspoons of butter or sprinkle with nonstick spray oil. Bake 1/3 layer of tortillas in the bottom of the pot and cover with baked bacon and 1/3 layer of cheese.

Place another third of the tortillas in the pan and cover with the cooked and chopped sausages and place another third of the cheese in layers.

Repeat with the last tortilla, ham and cheese 1/3. Mix eggs, milk, salt, pepper, garlic powder, and hot sauce. Pour the egg mixture evenly over the pot.

If desired, cover overnight and refrigerate or bake immediately. Set the oven to 350 degrees. Bake covered with foil for 45 minutes. Find and cook for another 20 minutes until the cheese is completely melted and cooked in a pan.

Nutrition: Calories 447 - Fat 32.6g - Carbohydrates 14.6g

Pecan-Banana Pops

Preparation Time: 10 minutes

Cooking Time: 15 minutes

Servings: 4

Ingredients

4 large just-ripe bananas

2 tablespoons raw honey

4 Popsicle sticks

3A cup chopped pecans

½ cup almond butter

Kitchen Equipment:

microwave

small bowl

baking sheet

wax paper or foil

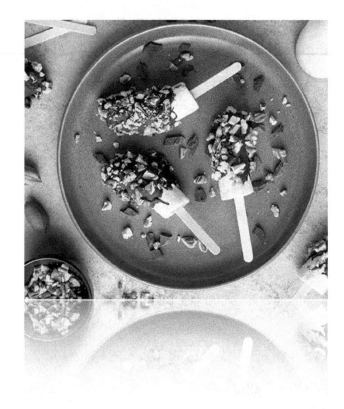

Directions:

Peel and cut one end from each banana, and insert a Popsicle stick into the cut end.

Combine together the almond butter and honey, and heat in the microwave for 10 to 15 seconds, or just until the mixture is slightly thinned. Pour onto a sheet of wax paper or aluminum foil and spread with a spatula.

On another piece of wax paper or foil, spread the chopped pecans — Line a small baking sheet or large plate with the third piece of wax paper or foil.

Roll each banana first in the honey mixture until well coated, then in the nuts until completely covered, pressing down gently, so the nuts adhere.

Place each finished banana onto the baking sheet. When all of the bananas have been coated, place the sheet in the freezer for at least 2 hours. For long-term storage, transfer the frozen bananas into a resealable plastic bag.

Nutrition: Fat 14g - Carbohydrates 7g - Protein14g

Greek Breakfast Wraps

Preparation Time: 10 minutes

Cooking Time: 15 minutes

Servings: 2

Ingredients

1 teaspoon olive oil

½ cup fresh baby spinach leaves

1 tablespoon fresh basil

4 egg whites, beaten

½ teaspoon salt

¼ teaspoon freshly ground black pepper

¼ cup crumbled low-fat feta cheese

2 (8-inch) whole-wheat tortillas

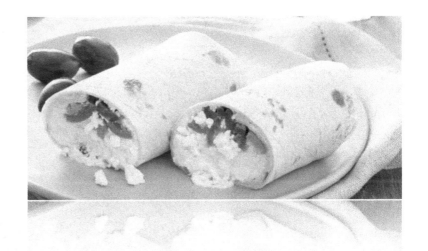

Kitchen Equipment:

small skillet

microwave

Directions:

Cook the olive oil over medium heat. Place the spinach and basil to the pan and sauté for about 2 minutes, or just until the spinach is wilted. Add the egg whites to the pan, season with the salt and pepper, and sauté, continue stirring until the egg whites are firm.

Turn off the heat and topped with the feta cheese. Warm up the tortillas until softened and warm in the microwave. Divide the eggs between the tortillas and wrap up burrito-style.

Nutrition: **Fat** 10.4g - **Carbohydrate** 4.5g - **Protein** 10.6g

Curried Chicken Breast Wraps

Preparation Time: 10 minutes

Cooking Time: 10 minutes

Servings: 2

Ingredients

6 ounces cooked chicken breast, cubed

1 small Gala or Granny Smith apple, cored and chopped

2 tablespoons plain low-fat yogurt

1 cup spring lettuce mix or baby lettuce

1 teaspoon Dijon mustard

½ teaspoon mild curry powder

2 (8-inch) whole-wheat tortillas

Kitchen Equipment:

Small bowl

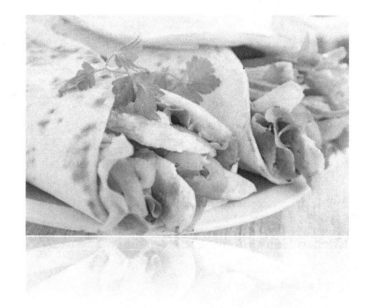

Directions:

Stir well the chicken, yogurt, Dijon mustard, and curry powder to combine. Add the apple and stir until blended.

Split the lettuce between the tortillas and top each with half of the chicken mixture. Roll up burrito-style and serve.

Nutrition:

Total fat 5g - **Carbohydrates** 18g - **Protein** 28g

Baked Salmon Fillets with Tomato and Mushrooms

Preparation Time: 10 minutes

Cooking Time: 20 minutes

Servings: 2

Ingredients

2 (4-ounce) skin-on salmon fillets

2 teaspoons olive oil, divided

½ teaspoon salt

¼ teaspoon freshly ground black pepper

½ teaspoon chopped fresh dill

½ cup diced fresh tomato

½ cup sliced fresh mushrooms

Kitchen Equipment:

oven

aluminum foil

pastry brush

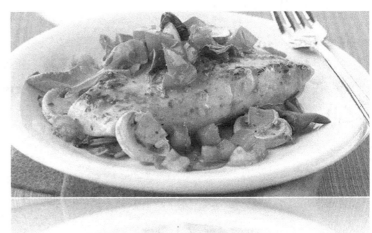

Directions:

Set the oven at 375 degrees and line a baking sheet with aluminum foil. You are using your fingers or a pastry brush, coat both sides of the fillets with ½ teaspoon of the olive oil each. Place the salmon skin-side down on the pan. Sprinkle salt and pepper equally all round.

In a small plate, mix the remaining 1 teaspoon olive oil, the tomato, mushrooms, and dill; stir well to combine. Spoon the mixture over the fillets.

Wrap it with foil to seal the fish, place the pan on the middle oven rack, and bake for about 20 minutes, or until the salmon flakes easily.

Nutrition: Fat 12.2g - **Carbohydrate** 21g - **Protein** 25.1g

Cinnamon and Spice Overnight Oats

Preparation Time: 10 minutes

Cooking Time: 0 minute

Servings: 1

Ingredients

75g rolled oats

100ml milk

75g yogurt

1 tsp. honey

1/2 tsp. vanilla extract

1/8th tsp. Schwartz ground cinnamon

20g raisins

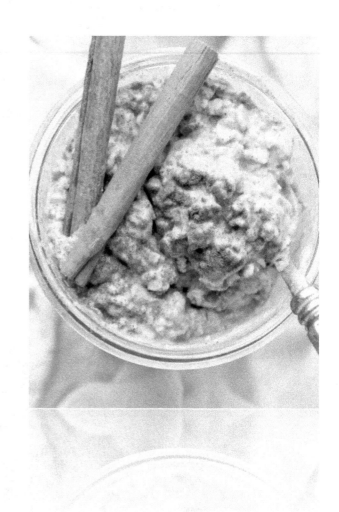

Kitchen Equipment:

bowl

microwave

Directions:

Incorporate all ingredients to a bowl and mix well. Cover overnight or at least one hour and refrigerate.

Exit the refrigerator or heat it in the microwave immediately or slowly.

Nutrition:

Carbohydrates 15g - **Protein** 26g - **Fat** 34g

Mexican Casserole

Preparation Time: 10 minutes

Cooking Time: 20 minutes

Servings: 6

Ingredients

1-pound lean ground beef

2 cups salsa

1 (16 ounces) can chili beans, drained

3 cups tortilla chips, crushed

2 cups sour cream

1 (2 ounces) can slice black olives, drained

1/2 cup chopped green onion

1/2 cup chopped fresh tomato

2 cups shredded Cheddar cheese

Kitchen Equipment:

oven

9x13 baking dish

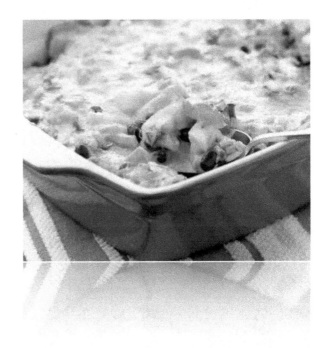

Directions:

Prepare oven to 350 degrees Fahrenheit (175 degrees Celsius).

In a large fish over medium heat, cook the meat so that it is no longer pink. Add the sauce, reduce the heat and simmer for 20 minutes or until the liquid is absorbed. Add beans and heat.

Sprinkle a 9x13 baking dish with oil spray. Pour the chopped tortillas into the pan and then place the meat mixture on it. Pour sour cream over meat and sprinkle with olives, green onions, and tomatoes. Top with cheddar cheese.

Bake in preheated oven for 30 minutes or until hot and bubbly.

Nutrition:

Fat 43.7 - **Carbohydrates** 32.8 - **Protein** 31.7g

Microwaved Fish and Asparagus with Tarragon Mustard Sauce

Preparation Time: 10 minutes

Cooking Time: 20 minutes

Servings: 2

Ingredients

12 ounces (340 g) fish fillets— whiting, tilapia, sole, flounder, or any kind of white fish

10 asparagus spears

2 tablespoons (30 g) sour cream

1 tablespoon (15 g) mayonnaise

¼ teaspoon dried tarragon

½ teaspoon Dijon or spicy brown mustard

Kitchen Equipment:

large plate

microwave

pie plate

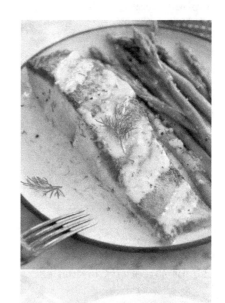

Directions:

Draw the bottom of the asparagus spears and cut them naturally. Put the asparagus on a large glass plate, add 1 teaspoon (15 ml) of water and cover with a plate. Microwave for 3 minutes.

While the asparagus is in the microwave, mix sour, mayonnaise, tarragon and mustard together.

Remove the asparagus from the microwave oven, remove it from the pie plate and set aside. Drain the water from the runway. Put the fish fillet in it

Peel the pie plate and spread 2 tablespoons (30 ml) cream mixture on them and cover the pie again and place the fish in the microwave for 3 to 4 minutes. Open the oven, remove the plate from the top of the pie plate and place the asparagus on top of the fish. Cover the pie plate again and cook for another 1-2 minutes.

Remove the pie plate from the microwave oven and remove the plate. Put the fish and asparagus on a serving platter. Chop any boiled sauce on a plate over fish and asparagus. Melt each with reserved sauce and serve.

Nutrition:

Carbs 4g - **Protein** 33g - **Fat** 17g

Keto pancakes

Preparation Time: 5 minutes

Cooking Time: 15 minutes

Servings: 10

Ingredients:

1/2 c. almond flour

4 oz. cream cheese softened

Four large eggs

1 tsp. lemon zest

Butter, for frying and serving

Kitchen Equipment:

nonstick skillet

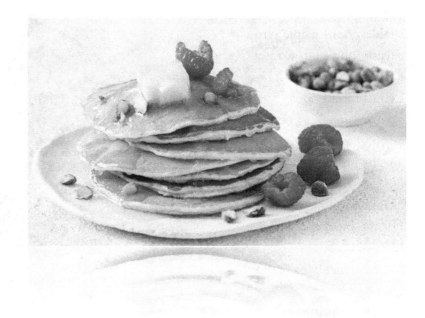

Directions:

Whisk almond flour, cream cheese, eggs, and lemon zest together in a medium bowl until smooth.

Heat one tablespoon butter over medium flame in a non-stick skillet. Pour in the batter for about three tablespoons, and cook for 2 minutes until golden. Flip over and cook for 2 minutes. Switch to a plate, and start with the batter remaining.

Serve with butter on top.

Nutrition:

calories 110

fats 10g

protein 28g

Greek Yogurt Fluffy Waffles

Preparation Time: 10 minutes

Cooking Time: 15 minutes

Servings: 5

Ingredients:

For the waffles:

1 cup Greek yogurt*

2 eggs whisked

2 tablespoons maple syrup

1 teaspoon vanilla extract

1 cup tapioca flour

1 cup almond flour

1 teaspoon baking powder

pinch of salt

For the toppings:

1/4 cup Greek yogurt*

1 tablespoon maple syrup

1/4 cup blueberries

1/4 cup blackberries

1/4 cup strawberries, diced

1/4 cup raspberries

Kitchen Equipment:

medium bowl

large bowl

scooper

Waffle iron

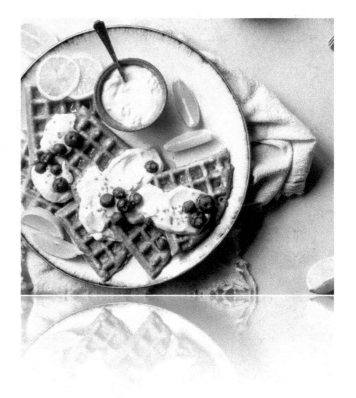

Directions:

Heat up waffle iron and oil it up. Whisk milk, eggs, maple syrup, yogurt, and the vanilla extract together in a medium bowl. Whisk the tapioca and almond flour, baking powder and salt together in a larger bowl. Add wet ingredients into dry elements and mix until well mixed.

Use an ice cream scoop to scoop in the greased waffle iron around ¼ cup of the batter and cook the waffle until it is cooked through inside and crispy outside. The batter will make roughly five-round waffles.

Once the waffles are fried, whisk the yogurt and the maple syrup together and cover each waffle with a spoonful of fruit on top!

Nutrition: Calories 120 - **Fats** 14g - **Protein** 31g

Light and Crispy Vanilla Protein Waffles

Preparation Time: 10 minutes

Cooking Time: 30 minutes

Servings: 4

Ingredients:

3/4 cup applesauce

4 eggs whisked

1 teaspoon vanilla extract

2 tablespoons coconut oil, melted

1 cup tapioca flour (or arrowroot powder)

1 cup Vanilla Primal Fuel protein

1 teaspoon baking soda

1/4 teaspoon cinnamon

pinch of salt

maple syrup, to garnish

coconut whipped cream, to garnish

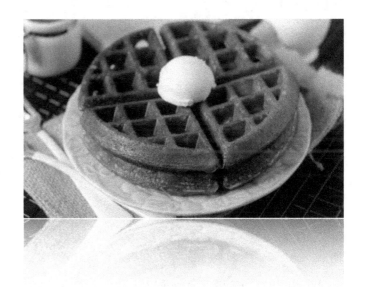

Kitchen Equipment:

waffle iron

Directions:

Whisk applesauce, milk, vanilla extract, and coconut oil together.

Add flour and whisk the tapioca until mixed. Then add protein powder to combine and whisk again. Eventually, add cinnamon, baking soda, and a pinch of salt and blend well.

Pour batter into the waffle iron and cook until crispy. It was taking less than 5 minutes for each waffle. Repeat with batter's rest.

Garnish with cream and maple syrup, whipped with coconut.

Nutrition: calories 117 - **fats** 9g - **protein** 27g

Hearty Hot Cereal with Berries

Preparation Time: 10 minutes

Cooking Time: 5 minutes

Servings: 4

Ingredients

4 cups of water

2 tablespoons honey

½ teaspoon salt

½ cup fresh blueberries

2 cups whole rolled oats

½ cup fresh raspberries

½ cup chopped walnuts

cup low-fat milk

teaspoons flaxseed

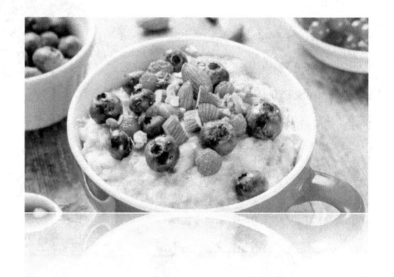

Kitchen Equipment:

Medium saucepan

Directions:

Boil water over high heat and stir in the salt in a medium saucepan. Stir in the oats, walnuts, and flaxseed, then reduce the heat to low and cover — Cook for 16 to 20 minutes, or until the oatmeal reaches the desired consistency.

Divide the oatmeal between 4 deep bowls and top each with 2 tablespoons of both blueberries and raspberries. Add ½ cup milk to each bowl and serve.

Nutrition: - **Fat** 15g - **Carbohydrates** 17g - **Protein** 19g

Protein Power Sweet Potatoes

Preparation Time: 15 minutes

Cooking Time: 10 minutes

Servings: 2

Ingredients

2 medium sweet potatoes

6 ounces plain Greek yogurt

½ teaspoon salt

1/3 cup dried cranberries

¼ teaspoon freshly ground black pepper

Kitchen Equipment:

oven

cooking plate

medium bowl

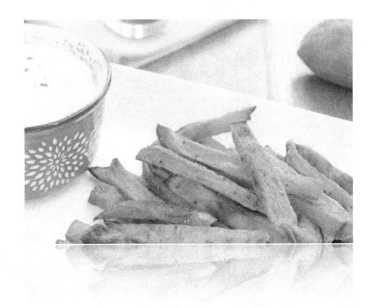

Directions:

Prepare the oven at 400 degrees F and prick the sweet potatoes several times. Place them on a cooking plate and cook for 40 to 45 minutes, or until you can easily pierce them with a fork.

Cut the potatoes in half and wrap the meat in a medium bowl and keep the skin healthy.

Add the salt, pepper, yogurt, and cranberries to the bowl and mix well with a fork.

Return the mixture back into the potato skins and serve warm.

Nutrition:

Fat 11g - **Carbohydrates** 15g - **Protein** 18g